Dental Caries - The Selection of Restoration Methods and Restorative Materials

Edited by Laura-Cristina Rusu and Lavinia Cosmina Ardelean

Published in London, United Kingdom

Dental Caries - The Selection of Restoration Methods and Restorative Materials
http://dx.doi.org/10.5772/intechopen.100795
Edited by Laura-Cristina Rusu and Lavinia Cosmina Ardelean

Contributors
Francisco Wanderley Garcia Paula-Silva, Luanna Gonçalves Ferreira, Giuliana de Campos Chaves Lamarque, Manal A. Ablal, Husniya Azim, Shiba Azim, Reghunathan Preethanath, Aiswarya Anil, Wael I. Ibraheem, Abdullah A. Meshni, Sukumaran Anil, Lavinia Cosmina Ardelean, Laura-Cristina Cristina Rusu, Alexandra Roi, Codruta Victoria Tigmeanu, Ciprian Ioan Roi, Atena Galuscan, Aurora Doris Fratila, Daniela Jumanca

First published in London, United Kingdom, 2022 by IntechOpen
IntechOpen is the global imprint of INTECHOPEN LIMITED, registered in England and Wales, registration number: 11086078, 5 Princes Gate Court, London, SW7 2QJ, United Kingdom

British Library Cataloguing-in-Publication Data
A catalogue record for this book is available from the British Library

Additional hard and PDF copies can be obtained from orders@intechopen.com

Dental Caries - The Selection of Restoration Methods and Restorative Materials
Edited by Laura-Cristina Rusu and Lavinia Cosmina Ardelean
p. cm.

This title is part of the Dentistry Book Series, Volume 12
Topic: Oral Health
Series Editor: Sergio Alexandre Gehrke
Topic Editor: Sandra Marinho and Esra Guzeldemir-Akcakanat

Print ISBN 978-1-80356-359-6
Online ISBN 978-1-80356-360-2
eBook (PDF) ISBN 978-1-80356-361-9
ISSN 2631-6218

IntechOpen Book Series

Dentistry

Volume 12

Aims and Scope of the Series

This book series will offer a comprehensive overview of recent research trends as well as clinical applications within different specialties of dentistry. Topics will include overviews of the health of the oral cavity, from prevention and care to different treatments for the rehabilitation of problems that may affect the organs and/or tissues present. The different areas of dentistry will be explored, with the aim of disseminating knowledge and providing readers with new tools for the comprehensive treatment of their patients with greater safety and with current techniques. Ongoing issues, recent advances, and future diagnostic approaches and therapeutic strategies will also be discussed. This series of books will focus on various aspects of the properties and results obtained by the various treatments available, whether preventive or curative.

Meet the Series Editor

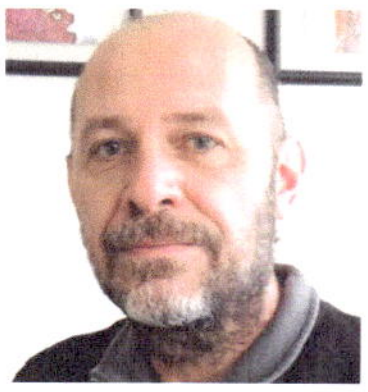

Dr. Sergio Alexandre Gehrke is a doctorate holder in two fields. The first is a Ph.D. in Cellular and Molecular Biology from the Pontificia Catholic University, Porto Alegre, Brazil, in 2010 and the other is an International Ph.D. in Bioengineering from the Universidad Miguel Hernandez, Elche/Alicante, Spain, obtained in 2020. In 2018, he completed a postdoctoral fellowship in Materials Engineering in the NUCLEMAT of the Pontificia Catholic University, Porto Alegre, Brazil. He is currently the Director of the Postgraduate Program in Implantology of the Bioface/UCAM/PgO (Montevideo, Uruguay), Director of the Cathedra of Biotechnology of the Catholic University of Murcia (Murcia, Spain), an Extraordinary Full Professor of the Catholic University of Murcia (Murcia, Spain) as well as the Director of the private center of research Biotecnos – Technology and Science (Montevideo, Uruguay). Applied biomaterials, cellular and molecular biology, and dental implants are among his research interests. He has published several original papers in renowned journals. In addition, he is also a Collaborating Professor in several Postgraduate programs at different universities all over the world.

Meet the Volume Editors

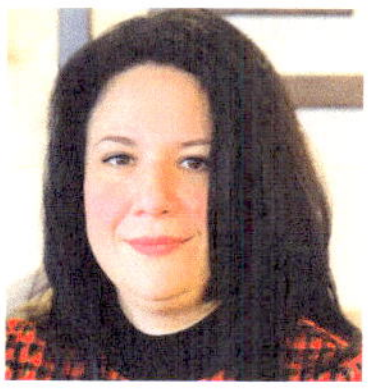

Professor Laura Cristina Rusu, DMD, Ph.D., is the mother of two lovely boys and a full-time professor and head of the Oral Pathology Department, Faculty of Dental Medicine, "Victor Babes" University of Medicine and Pharmacy, Timisoara, Romania. Her Ph.D. thesis was on allergens in dental materials. In 2017 she obtained a Dr. Habil and was confirmed as Ph.D. coordinator in dental medicine. She has taken part in ten research projects, including FP7 COST Action MP 1005. She has authored more than 140 peer-reviewed papers, nine books, and several book chapters and co-edited one book. She served as guest editor for four journal special issues. She currently holds two patents. Dr. Rusu is a member of the editorial board of the *Journal of Science and Arts* and *Medicine in Evolution*, a topic editor for *Materials*, and an academic editor for *Scanning*. Her main scientific interests are oral pathology and oral diagnosis in dental medicine, focusing on oral cancer.

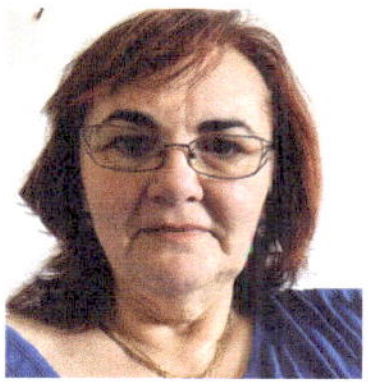

Professor Lavinia Cosmina Ardelean, DMD, Ph.D., is a professor and head of the Department of Technology of Materials and Devices in Dental Medicine, "Victor Babes" University of Medicine and Pharmacy, Timisoara, Romania. She has authored/co-authored 16 books, 11 book chapters, and more than 120 peer-reviewed papers. She has also edited one book. She is an editorial board member of numerous journals, a member of reviewer/topic boards for *Materials*, *Prosthesis*, *Metals*, *Polymers*, and *Journal of Functional Biomaterials*, and an academic editor for *Scanning*. She has served as guest editor for eight journal special issues. Being an active reviewer, with more than 200 reviews to her credit so far, Dr. Ardelean received the 2019 Top Reviewers in Cross-Field Award, and the 2019 Top Reviewers in Materials Science Award. She currently holds one patent. Her research interests include most areas of dentistry, with a focus on dental materials/biomaterials, dental alloys, resins, ceramics/bioceramics, CAD/CAM milling, 3D printing/bioprinting in dentistry, laser welding, scanning, and oral health care.

Contents

Preface

According to the World Health Organization (WHO), 2.3 billion people worldwide suffer from permanent teeth caries. The prevalence of primary teeth caries is estimated to be 530 million. Untreated dental caries is a common health condition, affecting people throughout their lifetime. Dental caries is an issue in modern society that is sometimes difficult to manage. Prevention and regular dental check-ups are of utmost importance in the proper management of caries, which, untreated, may result in oral pain, aesthetic impairment, and edentulism. They can also affect the adjoining oral tissues and potentially lead to systemic complications. Public health measures addressing risk factors as well as access to oral health services enable a successful approach to the management of dental caries. Lack of appropriate health facilities and limited access to primary oral health services is, unfortunately, still quite common in certain geographical areas. As high costs of dental treatment may represent a major barrier for large categories of people, targeted health programs and specific approaches are to be more broadly attempted to overcome these issues.

In cases where restorative treatment is needed, materials choice and proper handling as well as a selection of restorative methods are crucial in preventing the occurrence and recurrence of complications. The currently available dental materials are in constant development, and techniques such as lasers, microscopy, and 3D bioprinting are becoming more complex. New state-of-the-art restorative materials, such as antimicrobial composites, stimuli-responsive composites, or self-healing composites, together with the use of nanotechnology, represent some of the future choices for restorative biomaterials.

This book, consisting of seven chapters, focuses on different aspects of dental caries, including etiology, diagnosis, prevention, treatment, and management. The introductory chapter presents general considerations about dental caries. Subsequent chapters discuss the dynamics of demineralization and remineralization and their role in the etiology of dental caries, as well as the influence of salivary pH in the prevalence of dental caries. The book also examines the relationship between diet and nutrition with early childhood dental caries. Finally, the book discusses the management of caries using modern diagnostic approaches, such as fluorescence-based devices, and novel treatment techniques, including minimally invasive atraumatic restorative treatment.

Laura-Cristina Rusu
Department of Oral Pathology,
"Victor Babes" University of Medicine and Pharmacy Timisoara,
Timișoara, Romania

Lavinia Cosmina Ardelean
Department of Technology of Materials and Devices in Dental Medicine,
"Victor Babes" University of Medicine and Pharmacy Timisoara,
Timișoara, Romania

Chapter 1

Introductory Chapter: Dental Caries-General Considerations

Laura-Cristina Rusu and Lavinia Cosmina Ardelean

1. Introduction

Dental caries, a most common chronic disease, affecting the global population, has been defined as: "a biofilm-mediated, sugar-driven, multifactorial, dynamic disease that results in the phasic demineralization and remineralization of dental hard tissues" [1].

Dental caries is currently considered the most prevalent chronic oral disease, with great influence on both oral and systemic health, as oral bacteria play specific roles in secondary infections of internal organs, with potentially serious consequences on the general health [2].

2. Dental caries-general considerations

Dental caries is primarily caused by the interaction of the oral biofilm with fermentable dietary carbohydrates on the tooth surface, but its etiology is, in fact, much more complex, involving the influence of numerous risk and protective factors, as well [3].

Dental caries is represented by the localized demineralization of the tooth structure, with progressive loss of its components. The main process involved in its initiation is the demineralization of the tooth, in the presence of a low salivary pH, further exposing the dental structures to the action of pathological agents.

Being the first body fluid coming in contact with oral pathogens, saliva is responsible for their neutralization, thus controlling the homeostasis of the oral environment. The flow rate, composition, and pH of the saliva are important variables for the initiation and progression of dental caries. It also plays an important role in controlling the mineral content of the tooth and protecting its integrity, being involved in the remineralization process [4].

Dietary habits are another important factor in developing dental caries. A frequent exposure to fermentable carbohydrates triggers modifications of the oral environment, which facilitate the growth of acidogenic bacteria and appearance of cariogenic biofilm. A retentive tooth anatomy, with steep pits and fissures or with gingival recession, exposing the root, represents favoring factors [5].

Basically, the cumulative action of all these factors, for a certain period of time, results in occurrence of dental caries. Characterized by a progressive evolution, dental caries is being reversible in early stages of the demineralization process [6].

A proper oral hygiene is crucial in preventing or arresting the process. Tooth brushing, flossing, and rinsing not only mechanically clean the teeth, and disrupt the biofilm, but also remove most of the bacteria and enable new colonization of the clean tooth surface. In cases of high risk of developing dental caries, topical fluoride agents are frequently recommended as a preventive method. However, rough surfaces restrict proper biofilm removal. In cases of steep pits and fissures, sealants play an important role in preventing and arresting initial lesions [1].

Caries detection in early stages of demineralization, when only enamel has been affected, is traditionally carried out by visual inspection and probing, appearing as white, chalky, and opaque spots, with unaltered surface texture, in case of non-cavitated lesions. As the lesion advances, a rough surface, softer than sound enamel, can be detected. Noncavitated lesions on proximal surfaces are visually undetectable. A cavitated enamel lesion is perceived as a surface breakdown, sensitive to probing. After passing the dentin-enamel junction, the carious process advances more rapidly, spreading in the less mineralized dentin, weaker to the acid attack. In this stage, pain and sensitivity usually occur. With the aid of currently available detection methods, such as fluorescence-based or light-based techniques, early detection of caries has become handy [7].

When caries progresses, causing tooth structure destruction, it requires repair, the main goal is preserving the vitality of the pulp. Conservative preparations, followed by small-size restorations, have a potentially less negative impact on tooth function and esthetics, also preserving the strength of the remnant hard tissue.

Materials choice and selection have to consider several factors, and the dentist has to present the available choices to the patient. Usually, patient's decision is mainly focused on esthetic and price considerations, but, other important factors, such as the extent of the preparation and the possibility of proper isolation of the working field, should be taken into account.

The most common choice is composite restorations, adhesively bonded, which allow a conservative approach to the preparation, and also provide excellent esthetics [8].

However, untreated dental caries may result in complications, usually accompanied by severe pain, with an important impact on daily living. The ultimate consequences are acute or chronic pulpitis and apical periodontitis, which require much more complicated and expensive treatment. Extreme cases may even require tooth extraction, followed by undesired repercussions on local and general health.

3. Conclusion

The goal in the management of dental caries is to address its causative factors, and maintain a neutral oral pH.

Conflict of interest

The authors declare no conflict of interest.

Author details

Laura-Cristina Rusu[1] and Lavinia Cosmina Ardelean[2*]

1 Department of Oral Pathology, Multidisciplinary Center for Research, Evaluation, Diagnosis and Therapies in Oral Medicine, "Victor Babes" University of Medicine and Pharmacy, Timisoara, Romania

2 Department of Technology of Materials and Devices in Dental Medicine, Multidisciplinary Center for Research, Evaluation, Diagnosis and Therapies in Oral Medicine, "Victor Babeş" University of Medicine and Pharmacy, Timisoara, Romania

*Address all correspondence to: lavinia_ardelean@umft.ro

References

[1] Caries Risk Assessment and Management. 2021. Available from: https://www.ada.org/resources/research/science-and-research-institute/oral-health-topics/caries-risk-assessment-and-management. [Accessed: August 26, 2022]

[2] Kim JK, Baker LA, Davarian S, Crimmins E. Oral health problems and mortality. Journal of Dental Science. 2013;**8**:10.1016. DOI: 10.1016/j.jds.2012.12.011], 10.1016/j.jds.2012.12.011]

[3] Ritter AV, Scott Eidson R, Donovan TE. Dental caries: Etiology, clinical characteristics, risk assessment, and management. In: Heyman HO, Swift EJ, Ritter AV, editors. Sturdevant's Art and Science of Operative Dentistry. 6th ed. Amsterdam, The Netherlands: Elsevier; 2014. pp. 41-88

[4] Vellore G, Arzreanne AR. Saliva as a diagnostic tool for assessment of dental caries. Archives of Orofacial Sciences. 2006;**1**:57-59

[5] Ferreira Zandona AG, Ritter AV, Eidson RS. Dental caries: Etiology, clinical characteristics, risk assessment, and management. In: Ritter AV, Boushell LW, Walter R, editors. Sturdevant's Art and Science of Operative Dentistry. 7th ed. Amsterdam, The Netherlands: Elsevier; 2018. pp. 40-94

[6] Jepsen S, Blanco J, Buchalla W, Carvalho JC, Dietrich T, Dorfer T, et al. Prevention and control of dental caries and periodontal diseases at individual andpopulation level: Consensus report of group 3 of joint EFP/ORCA workshop on the boundaries between caries and periodontal diseases. Journal of Clinical Periodontology. 2017;**44**(Suppl. 44):S85-S93. DOI: 10.1111/jcpe.12687

[7] Gomez J. Detection and diagnosis of the early caries lesion. BMC Oral Health. 2015;**15**(Suppl. 1):S3. DOI: 10.1186/1472-6831-15-S1-S3

[8] Tooth Cavities. 2017. Available from: https://www.healthline.com/find-care/articles/dentists/tooth-cavities. [Accessed: August 26, 2022]

Chapter 2

Demineralization and Remineralization Dynamics and Dental Caries

Aiswarya Anil, Wael I. Ibraheem, Abdullah A. Meshni, Reghunathan Preethanath and Sukumaran Anil

Abstract

Dental caries is a multifactorial disease caused by the interaction of dietary sugars, dental biofilm, and the dental tissue of the host. It results from repeated cycles of demineralization and remineralization at the interface of the biofilm and the tooth surface. Demineralization is the process of removing mineral ions from hydroxyapatite crystals in hard tissues, such as enamel, which can lead to dental caries if left unchecked. The remineralization process can reverse the lost mineral ions that occur during demineralization. The degree of demineralization and remineralization depends on several variables, including the amount of available calcium and phosphate and salivary pH levels. Over the past several decades, remineralizing or calcifying fluids with variable calcium, phosphate, and fluoride formulations have been developed. The management of early caries by remineralization has the potential to significantly advance the noninvasive clinical management of the disease. The chapter outlines the mechanisms by which the demineralization-remineralization process occurs and the use of remineralizing agents that reverse demineralization or enhance remineralization.

Keywords: demineralization, enamel, white lesions, remineralization, dentistry, dental caries

1. Introduction

Dental caries is one of the most significant public health issues and a highly prevalent disease worldwide. It is an irreversible, chronic, infectious disease that progresses as a dynamic, multifactorial process and affects the mineralized dental structures. Dental caries is a complex disease caused by the demineralization and remineralization of enamel in the presence of fermentable carbohydrates, saliva, and cariogenic oral flora. When exposed to carbohydrates, oral microorganisms can produce organic acids that lower the pH of dental plaque. Caries progresses through demineralization and remineralization phases on the tooth surface before invading deeper layers [1].

Enamel consists of hydroxyapatite, water, protein, and trace elements, such as fluoride. The organic matrix consists of noncollagenous protein, amelogenin, and inorganic components consists of enamel's biological apatite. Enamel apatite has a hexagonal unit cell composed of prismatic crystals and contains more inorganic material than dentin, bone, and cementum [2]. Twenty percent of a tooth's matrix consists of organic material, which makes up the majority of the tooth's dentine. Most of the organic portion of dentine comprises Type I collagen, while the remainder consists of collagen types III and V [3]. The surface layer of enamel is composed of hydroxyapatite (HA) crystals that form the prism of enamel. HA is a crystalline form of calcium (CA++), hydroxyl (OH), and phosphate ions (PO43−) that compose the mineral structure of bones and teeth. The surface layer's hardness is primarily the result of a high concentration of phosphate ions, fluorine, calcium, and chlorine. Enamel adjacent to dentine is softer due to its high magnesium, sodium, and potassium ion content [1, 4].

2. Demineralization

Demineralization refers to the process by which organic acids produced by plaque microorganisms destroy the mineral content from the surface of HA crystals. The most stable form of hydroxyapatite exists in an environment with a pH of 7.4. There is a constant chemical equilibrium between the hydroxyapatite in the enamel (Ca10(PO4)6(OH)2) and the dissolved hydroxyapatite in the plaque biofilm. Mineral crystal dissolution takes place when the pH level of the plaque falls below 5.5 [5, 6]. When the minerals are dissolved, the intercrystalline space expands, and the surface of the enamel becomes softer and more porous, leading to the formation of caries [6]. Due to the acid metabolism of cariogenic microorganisms in dental plaque biofilm, enamel demineralization occurs (**Figure 1**). The greatest degree of demineralization in enamel caries occurs at a subsurface level covered by a surface layer that appears relatively unaffected by the attack. This means that the majority of the mineral loss during the initial stages of demineralization occurs at a distance away from the enamel surface. This subsurface lesion is commonly referred to as "white spot lesions," which refers to an opaque white area that can be distinguished from healthy enamel. This stage of the carious lesion is visible as a white spot (WS) during a routine dental clinical examination and is known as initial caries, which can turn brown due to the absorption of pigments into enamel pores.

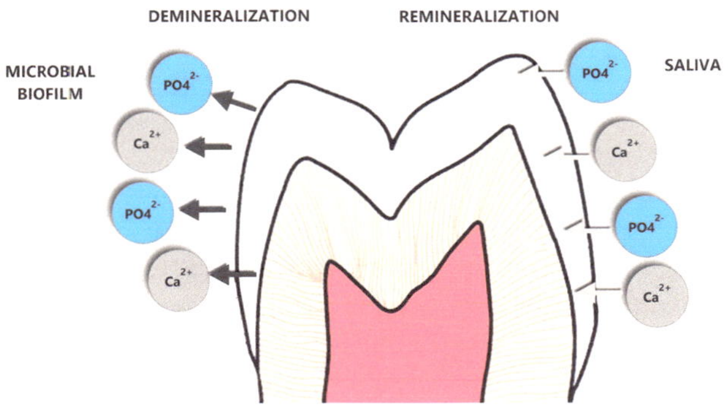

Figure 1.
Diagrammatic representation showing the equilibrium between dynamic demineralization and remineralization at the plaque-enamel interface. Saliva is a source of mineral and fluoride ions that promote remineralization of lesions.

Earlier *in vitro* experiments using organic acid buffers as demineralizing media explained the presence of the unaltered surface enamel resistant to acid dissolution by adsorption of organic matter onto the enamel crystallites [1, 7, 8]. Later studies recognized the reprecipitation process with respect to saturation of calcium and phosphates occurring at the underlying enamel layer [9–11]. According to *in vivo* microscopic studies, a mineral loss is initiated in the interprismatic regions and later proceeds into the enamel prisms [12, 13]. However, under oral conditions enamel demineralization is affected by a number of factors, such as modification in the microbial activity and changes in the physicochemical properties of the enamel mineral content. Studies using a polarizing microscope revealed that the porous subsurface enamel is positively birefringent, whereas the surface zone retains its negative birefringence [14, 15]. This indicates that the subsurface enamel has a demineralized zone with a pore volume greater than 25%, whereas the surface enamel has a pore volume less than 5% [16].

3. Remineralization

Remineralization occurs as a process of restoring minerals in the form of mineral ions to the hydroxyapatite latticework structure. Remineralization is a natural repair process for non-cavitated lesions that utilizes calcium and phosphate ions to construct a new surface on existing crystal remnants in subsurface lesions that remain after demineralization. These acid-resistant remineralized crystals are considerably less soluble than the original mineral. The major protein in dentine is predominantly type I collagen, which constitutes 90% of the organic matrix. They provide a scaffold for the deposition of minerals in dentine remineralization. Earlier studies were based on ion-mediated crystallization [17, 18] where epitaxial growth occurs over existing apatite crystallites within the demineralized collagen matrix. Although *in vitro* studies with a solution containing calcium and phosphorus ions induced calcium phosphate crystal deposition on the collagen surface, other studies with a solution containing fluoride and mineral ions showed better dentine remineralization [19–21].

4. Modifying factors/variables

These variables may be intrinsic or extrinsic. Diet and medication are examples of extrinsic factors, whereas intrinsic factors are the underlying systemic diseases. Physicochemical changes in enamel surface are also affected by behavior (frequency of tooth brushing and consumption of soft drinks) and socioeconomic status. Modifiable behavioral factors include the types of drinks consumed, the method of drinking, and the frequency of drinking [22]. Several medications cause xerostomia by decreasing salivary flow and pH, thereby diminishing the buffering effect against endogenous and exogenous acids [23, 24]. Intrinsic factors, such as gastroesophageal reflux disease and bulimia nervosa, cause demineralization and erosion of tooth enamel. The pH of endogenous acids is below the critical pH for HA dissolution, resulting in demineralized enamel surface areas [25, 26]. These regions may eventually harbor acid-forming bacteria, resulting in caries formation [27, 28].

5. White spot lesions

The earliest visible symptom caused by the demineralization of enamel is the appearance of white spots. Here, the actual demineralization affects the subsurface layer, while the surface of enamel remains smooth. This defect in the enamel is due to modifications of the chemical composition of the substrate. The translucency of enamel depends on the presence of water around prisms. Demineralization causes the widening of interprismatic space, and the water gets replaced by air. The light scattering effect occurs when there is a difference in refractive index between the two phases. The refractive index of healthy enamel is the same as that of hydroxyapatite (1.62) and therefore, there are no interfaces in healthy enamel (**Figure 2**). In hypo-mineralized enamel, light passes through mineral and fluid phases with different refractive indices, resulting in a white optical phenomenon seen as a "white spot" on the enamel surface. During the initial phase, the surface of a tooth has to be dried up in order to see a carious lesion. Microscopic studies report that if the white spot appears only after the tooth surface was dried up with air, the lesion is small, whereas if it is visible even without drying, it means the lesion is more advanced [29, 30].

The first stages of the carious disease are characterized by hypomineralization without cavity formation and are referred to as white spots (WS). During the initial carious formation, alternating phases of demineralization and remineralization cause the dissolution of mineral salts followed by reprecipitation of minerals on the enamel surface. This results in an intact surface layer, under which the body of the carious lesion extends in a half-moon shape or "cone shape" toward the demineral-ization zone [31]. The surface layer resembling healthy enamel is usually 20–50 μm deep. Hypomineralization of the subsurface causes enlargement of the enamel pores leading to mineral dissolution [32]. The central layer or body of the lesion is the most affected with 5% mineral loss in the peripheral part to 25% in the central part. The lesion becomes clinically visible when the mineral deficit in this layer compared to healthy enamel reaches 10%. The dark zone at the advancing front of the lesion is considered as a breakdown stage successional to the translucent zone and preceding the body of the lesion. *In vitro* studies [33, 34] reported large pores in the translucent zone, whereas in the dark zones, a micropore system is found in addition to the large

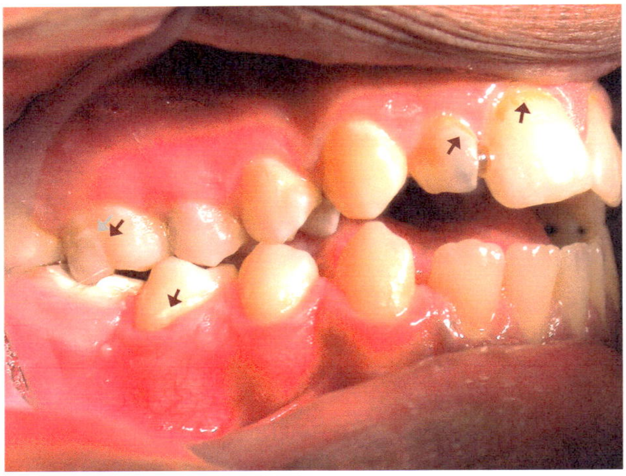

Figure 2.
White spot lesions after orthodontic treatment with fixed appliances.

pores, which was explained as areas of demineralization. The deeper translucent layer is seen close to healthy enamel and its occurrence is the first symptom of the pathological process [29]. *In vitro* studies on human enamel revealed the physical and chemical properties of surface enamel [35, 36]. One probability is the reprecipitation of calcium and phosphate ions released by subsurface dissolution or from the saturated solution in plaque biofilm into the surface enamel. The presence of fluoride ions in the surface enamel also helps in maintaining the surface zone from demineralization [33].

6. Dental caries

Dental caries is a cavity that forms on the tooth surface in the form of a small lesion that progresses and results in the loss of tooth structure (**Figure 3**). Demineralization causes initial changes at the ultrastructural level, which can only be observed with an electron microscope. Clinically, it cannot be detected in its earliest stages, but as the disease progresses, the dentist will notice a decrease in the enamel's translucency, which can be detected during an intraoral examination of the patient. When bacteria accumulate in dental plaque and ferment dietary carbohydrates for an extended period of time and the locally produced acids cannot be neutralized by the buffering capacity of saliva, demineralization of the teeth occurs, leading to cavities [37]. Although the ability of low pH to demineralize enamel is well-established [38, 39], dental caries is a multifactorial disease caused by microbes and influenced by dietary habits, tooth characteristics, saliva-buffering capacity, and host immune system [40].

The highly organized pellicle-covered dental plaque biofilm on the tooth surface contains live and dead bacterial cells, end products, desquamated epithelial cells, leukocytes, and glycoproteins from saliva. Cariogenic microorganisms metabolize carbohydrates from food to produce organic acid, primarily lactic or acetic acid. Dental caries initiates with surface roughness or subsurface demineralization, later progressing to cavitation. Initial studies indicated the presence of acidogenic

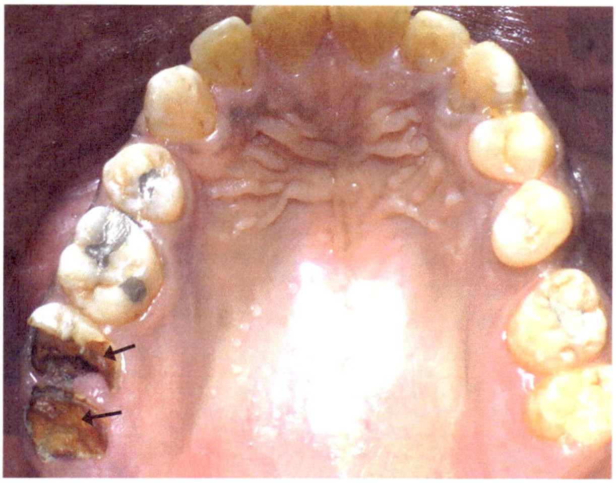

Figure 3.
Dental caries leads to the destruction of tooth structures.

streptococci mutans in dental caries [41, 42], and later lactobacilli species were also proposed to produce acid that causes dental caries [43, 44]. *In vitro* studies on bacterial species in caries lesions using PCR and specific DNA probes [45, 46] indicated that dental cavities are a complex ecosystem containing multiple cariogenic bacterial species, such as Veillonella or Corynebacterium [47].

Saliva mechanically cleanses the tooth surface of bacteria and food particles. Saliva's composition and secretion also play a significant role in demineralization. Calcium and phosphorus, the inorganic components of saliva, contribute to maintaining the mineral balance between hydroxyapatite of enamel and saliva. If the acid metabolites of microbes are not neutralized by the buffering properties of saliva, the pH of dental plaque decreases, thereby fostering demineralization of enamel. To preserve tooth structure, it is essential to maintain a balance between demineralization and remineralization of enamel [48].

7. Role of saliva in demineralization and remineralization process

A variety of oral and systemic factors can have a positive or negative effect on the constant cycle of demineralization/remineralization processes. Assessing patients' caries risk and recommending appropriate remineralization therapies for those deemed at high risk is critical for improving their oral health. Saliva is a critical factor in determining caries risk and remineralization. It is a critical biological and protective factor in the process of enamel remineralization [49]. The buffering capacity and secretion flow of saliva are proportional to the rate and extent of demineralization. Saliva can neutralize acids, form a protective membrane on tooth surfaces, and promote remineralization by providing enamel and dentin with calcium, phosphate, and fluoride [50]. The pH level of saliva directly affects remineralization through the amount of calcium and phosphate ions available to the enamel via saliva in times of acidic challenge [51]. Saliva can act as a replenishing agent and inhibit tooth demineralization during periods of low pH, while simultaneously promoting tooth remineralization once the pH returns to a neutral state. Systemic diseases, inherited disorders, a variety of medications, and other medical interventions can all have a detrimental effect on salivary production, buffering capacity, and the amount of calcium and phosphate available for remineralization [52, 53].

Saliva's protective properties are volume dependent. These protective properties can be significantly enhanced or diminished based on the rate of secretion in unstimulated and stimulated conditions. Unstimulated, normal salivary secretion is greater than 0.3 ml/minute, ranging between 0.5 and 1.5 L per day, compared to 0.1–0.7 ml/minute in patients with decreased salivary production [50]. Demineralization causes the loss of mineral ions, but it is reversible via remineralization. Both processes occur on the surface of the tooth, but cavitation necessitates a substantial loss of mineral ions from hydroxyapatite. A number of factors, including the availability of calcium and phosphate ions and the pH of the saliva, determine the degree of demineralization and remineralization. Individuals with decreased salivary flow have more acidic saliva and biofilm, which increases the risk of additional demineralization [54]. Reduced salivary flow also creates an oral environment that is unable to neutralize acids effectively, resulting in prolonged increase in intraoral pH [55]. The remineralization process is frequently hampered in patients with decreased salivary production, and the use of fluoride may be limited due to a deficiency of calcium and phosphate ions [56]. Fluoride, calcium, and phosphate are necessary for remineralization following a cariogenic attack. The focus of remineralization is mainly on detecting early caries lesions when the disease is still reversible. This helps in identifying the patients at risk. Saliva, fluoride therapy, and probiotic bacteria are considered as common regimes for tooth remineralization [57, 58].

8. Remineralizing agents

Several topical remineralizing agents have been used to inhibit and remineralize enamel (**Table 1**). For decades, fluoride has been the cornerstone of enamel remineralization. It is known to prevent caries by inhibiting demineralization on the surface of the enamel through the formation of fluorapatite. Fluorapatite is less soluble than hydroxyapatite and increases the enamel's resistance to dissolution during the acid attack. Varnishes, toothpastes, mouth rinses, solutions, gels, and orthodontic adhesives containing a fluoride source have been utilized as methods and formulations for fluoride delivery [59, 60].

8.1 Fluoride

The most common remineralizing agent is fluoride. When acid attacks the enamel surface, the pH begins to rise, and the presence of fluoride in the microenvironment stops enamel dissolution. As pH increases, new and larger fluoride crystals containing fluorhydroxyapatite form, reducing enamel demineralization and promoting remineralization [61, 62]. The fluoride acts on the enamel in several ways [61]. In the first mechanism, fluorapatite crystals have greater resistance to acid attack than hydroxyapatite crystals, which inhibits demineralization. Second, the combination of calcium and phosphate ions promotes remineralization by accelerating the formation of new fluorapatite crystals. It inhibits acid-producing carious bacteria by interfering with the synthesis of phosphoenol pyruvate, a crucial intermediate in the glycolytic

Compounds increasing mineral saturation
Fluorides
Casein phosphopeptide–amorphous calcium phosphate (CPP-ACP)
Bioactive glass
Tricalcium phosphate (TCP)
Nano HAP particles
Beta tricalcium phosphate (TCP)
Biofilm modifiers
Arginine
Triclosan
Xylitol
Probiotics
Herbal compounds

Table 1.
The remineralizing and biofilm modifying agents.

pathway of bacteria. In addition, fluoride adheres to oral hard tissue, oral mucosa, and dental plaque, thereby preventing demineralization and promoting remineralization. Fluoride concentrations on the surface of teeth can increase resistance to dental caries and erosion. In contrast, numerous laboratory studies have demonstrated that low levels of fluoride, such as those detected after many hours in resting plaque and saliva and resulting from daily use of fluoride dentifrices, have a significant impact on enamel demineralization and remineralization. Fluoride in the mouth affects the natural dissolution and reprecipitation processes that occur at the interface between the tooth and oral fluid. Trace amounts of fluoride accelerate the remineralization of early carious lesions [63, 64]. Stannous fluoride contains both fluoride and stannous ions, which possess antibacterial properties. It is also capable of forming stannous phosphate fluoride precipitates, which halt the progression of caries but discolor the teeth. The most effective technique for remineralization of early caries was twice-daily use of a 0.5% NaF mouth rinse in conjunction with twice-daily use of fluoride toothpaste. These findings suggest that the efficacy of fluoride is determined by the frequency of rinsing and the ability of the fluoride mouth rinse to reach inaccessible areas, such as interproximal spaces [65].

Studies have shown that fluoride released from a glass-ionomer restoration inhibits bacterial acid production by incorporating it into the biofilm of plaque bacteria [66, 67], in the adjacent tooth enamel and saliva of patients. Conventional and resin-modified glass ionomer can be recharged from external sources, such as topical fluoride application. Compared to resin-modified glass ionomers, glass ionomers emit comparatively greater amounts of fluorides. For effective remineralization, the fluoride release must be maintained at approximately 2–3 g/mL per day; this can be accomplished through fluoride recharge. Micro porosities present in conventional and resin-modified glass ionomers may account for the recharging capacity of these materials [67]. Pit-and-fissure sealants commonly used in preventive dentistry consist of either resin- or glass-ionomer-based materials. They prevent bacteria from settling in deep pits and fissures, thereby playing an important role in preventing dental caries. The incorporation of fluorides into sealant fillers promotes remineralization [23].

Dentifrices containing fluoride are regarded as the most effective agents for preventing enamel demineralization. Studies have demonstrated the effectiveness of conventional toothpastes containing 1000 ppm fluoride and the evidence suggests that toothpaste containing 5000 ppm fluoride can further reduce demineralization and enhance remineralization [68].

8.2 Casein phosphopeptide: amorphous calcium phosphate

Casein, a milk-derived protein developed by Eric Reynolds, mainly interacts with calcium and phosphate. They are used alone or as CPP-ACP (casein phosphopeptides with amorphous calcium phosphate) or CPP-ACFP (casein phosphopeptides with amorphous calcium fluoride phosphate). CPP-ACP is a two-phase system that precipitates onto the tooth structure and elevates calcium levels in the plaque biofilm and tooth enamel. CPP stabilizes ACP, maintaining a state of supersaturation of calcium and phosphate. As the pH of the material increases, the bound form of amorphous calcium phosphate also increases, thereby facilitating remineralization. The incorporation of casein phosphopeptide–amorphous calcium phosphate (CCP-ACP) into sealants facilitates the release of supersaturated levels of calcium and phosphate ions, which promotes the formation of new hydroxyapatite crystals and the remineralization of enamel subsurface lesions [69]. The advantage of CPPACFP is the availability of calcium, phosphate, and fluoride in one product, which can bind up to 25 calcium ions, 15 phosphate ions, and five fluoride ions, which helps in the remineralization of subsurface lesions in enamel [70–72]. Studies have shown CPP–ACP incorporated fluoride to a level of 900 ppm in toothpastes, chewing gum, lozenges, and mouth rinses give additive effects in reducing caries [73, 74]. Another in situ study with chewing gum containing CPP-ACP also showed a significant increase in mineral precipitation of initial bovine enamel lesions [75]. A study by Walker et al. [76] reported that the addition of CPP-ACP to milk resulted in enhanced remineralization.

8.3 Bioactive glass

Bioactive glass is a multi-component inorganic compound composed of sodium, calcium, phosphorus, and silica (sodium-calcium phosphosilicate). It helps in the formation of hydroxycarbonateapatite (HCA) crystals when it comes into contact with water, saliva, or other body fluids [72]. It has low cytotoxicity for dental pulp cells and exerts remineralization effects on both enamel and dentin. Additionally, its antimicrobial activity against intraoral bacteria has been established. It demonstrated the ability to neutralize acid and absorb calcium (Ca) ions in physiological conditions via its functional groups. It is a promising remineralization agent due to its biomimetic mineralizing properties. NovaMin®, a product of NovaMin Technology Inc. (NTI) available in the market containing bioactive glass and calcium sodium phosphosilicate has antimicrobial activity toward *Streptococcus mutans* (*S. mutans*) and *S. sanguis,* and also helps in the remineralization of tooth [77].

8.4 Tricalcium phosphate (TCP)

A new remineralizing agent, tricalcium phosphate is incorporated in dentifrices, which release calcium, phosphate, and fluoride when it comes in contact with the enamel surface during tooth brushing [73]. Functionalized TCP is a low-dose calcium phosphate system that is incorporated into a single-phase aqueous or non-aqueous topical fluoride formulation, which facilitates a targeted delivery of TCP when applied to the teeth. Studies have shown that the combination of TCP with fluoride can provide greater enamel remineralization and more acid-resistant mineral than fluoride alone [73].

8.5 Xylitol

The application of xylitol, a sugar alcohol of the pentitol type, on a regular basis has been linked to a marked reduction in caries and tooth remineralization. Xylitol is a nonfermentable sugar alcohol that has been demonstrated to have both noncariogenic and cariostatic properties. Xylitol interferes with the growth and metabolism of *S. mutans* by inhibiting glycolysis in the mitochondria of these microorganisms. Due to the inability of caries-causing bacteria to ferment xylitol, the acid attack is diminished when xylitol is consumed. As a result, the growth of these bacteria and the concurrent production of acid are inhibited, and the oral pH remains elevated. At high pH, the hydrophilic molecule of xylitol can form complexes with calcium in solution, thereby stabilizing the calcium and phosphates present in saliva. The saturation of calcium ions in saliva stimulates the remineralization of dental tissues through calcium ion deposition [78].

Xylitol increases salivary clearance, buffering capacity, and calcium and phosphate saturation by neutralizing the decreased plaque pH/salivary pH. Increased salivary flow increases acid buffering capacity, and the high mineral content helps in the remineralization of the damaged enamel [78]. There are conflicting reports about the effectiveness of xylitol, especially when taken with fluoride. Fluoride varnish, which contains xylitol-coated calcium and phosphate, released 10 times more fluoride in the first 4 hours than other varnishes like Enamel Pro® (Premier Dental Products, PA, USA) and Duraphat® (Colgate Oral Care, NSW, Australia) [79].

8.6 Arginine

Arginine is a semi-essential amino acid found in various proteins and peptides in human saliva. Non-pathogenic bacteria, such as *Streptococcus sanguinis*, utilize the arginine deiminase system to generate energy, ammonia, and carbon dioxide. The production of ammonia raises the local pH and neutralizes the acidifying effects of sugar metabolism, thereby promoting a more alkaline environment that is unfavorable to cariogenic bacteria and reducing the carcinogenicity of oral biofilms. Research has confirmed that arginine can affect the pH and ecology of oral biofilms. Therefore, it was added to toothpaste (1.5% arginine) containing insoluble calcium and 1450 ppm sodium monofluorophosphate in order to enhance caries lesion prevention via enhanced remineralization [80]. A systematic review concluded that this formulation possesses the potential for a superior anticaries effect [81]. Clinical studies have revealed that the new arginine-containing compound provided significantly greater benefits than conventional fluoride toothpaste alone in halting and reversing caries lesions [82, 83].

8.7 Triclosan

Triclosan is an antibacterial agent that may influence biofilm production, resulting in increased saturation and remineralization. Triclosan binds to bacterial cells and increases the permeability of the cells. High bactericidal concentrations induce membrane lesions that allow cellular content to leak out. There is a linear correlation between acid production inhibition and triclosan adsorption by *S. mutans* cells. Consequently, the effect of triclosan is not dependent on the concentration of triclosan in solution, but rather on the ratio between the amount of triclosan and the number of cells to be inhibited [84]. Studies conducted have demonstrated that the addition of triclosan to toothpaste formulations can result in modest but statistically significant reductions of coronal and root caries [85]. Silva et al. [86] suggested that it could also have an effect on remineralization.

8.8 Probiotics

WHO defined probiotic bacteria as "live microorganisms which, when administered in adequate amounts, confer a health benefit on the host" [87]. Probiotics is the idea of exploiting "good" bacteria to promote health. The concept is based on the theory of maintaining a healthy flora, which helps in eliminating pathogenic microbiota. Lactobacillus and Bifidobacterium, which are part of normal oral flora, are common examples of probiotics with oral health benefits used in the treatment of dental caries and periodontal disease by reducing the quantity of pathogenic bacteria or inhibiting the virulence genes of *S. mutans* [88, 89].

8.9 Herbal compounds

Several herbal and other natural compounds have been investigated as potential remineralization agents. Depending on the specific compound, they may influence mineral saturation and precipitation, act as antimicrobials, or stabilize collagen, which may serve as a scaffold for mineral deposition. Proanthocyanidins and calcium phosphate-based compounds may have a synergistic effect when remineralizing *in vitro* artificial root caries lesions [90]. Ginger rhizome (*Zingiber officinale Roscoe, Zingiberaceae*) and rosemary (*Rosmarinus officinalis L., Lamiaceae*) are antimicrobial herbs derived from natural food sources. In addition, they exhibit no toxicity. Several polyphenolic ketones with multiple pharmacological activities are present in the pungent oils of these herbs. Studies documented their antifungal and antimicrobial effects on oral cavity pathogens [91, 92]. Honey is a possible antibacterial agent, and research indicates that manuka honey is probably noncariogenic [93].

An *in vitro* study revealed that the application of ginger, honey, and rosemary as herbal medicines inhibited demineralization and promoted remineralization of enamel [94].

9. Conclusions

Several topical remineralizing agents have been used to inhibit and remineralize enamel and white spot lesions specifically. For decades, fluoride has been the cornerstone of enamel remineralization. It is known to prevent caries by inhibiting demineralization on the surface of the enamel through the formation of fluorapatite. Currently, new mineralization agents have been developed to preserve enamel integrity and prevent the formation of carious cavities. Modern dentistry focuses on managing non-cavitated caries lesions noninvasively via remineralization in order to prevent disease progression and improve esthetics, strength, and function. The evidence suggests that initial non-cavitated lesions can be remineralized using appropriate technologies, and even non-fluoride remineralization strategies.

Conflict of interest

The authors declare no conflict of interest.

Author details

Aiswarya Anil[1], Wael I. Ibraheem[2], Abdullah A. Meshni[2], Reghunathan Preethanath[2*] and Sukumaran Anil[3,4]

1 Saveetha Dental College, Saveetha Institute of Medical and Technical Sciences, Chennai, India

2 College of Dentistry, Jazan University, Jazan, Saudi Arabia

3 Department of Dentistry, Oral Health Institute, Hamad Medical Corporation, Doha, Qatar

4 College of Dental Medicine, Qatar University, Doha, Qatar

*Address all correspondence to: drpreethanath@gmail.com

References

[1] Abou Neel EA, Aljabo A, Strange A, Ibrahim S, Coathup M, Young AM, et al. Demineralization-remineralization dynamics in teeth and bone. International Journal of Nanomedicine. 2016;**11**:4743-4763

[2] Bigi A, Boanini E. Functionalized biomimetic calcium phosphates for bone tissue repair. Journal of Applied Biomaterials and Functional Materials. 2017;**15**(4):e313-e325

[3] Depalle B, McGilvery CM, Nobakhti S, Aldegaither N, Shefelbine SJ, Porter AE. Osteopontin regulates type I collagen fibril formation in bone tissue. Acta Biomaterialia. 2021;**120**:194-202

[4] Lacruz RS, Habelitz S, Wright JT, Paine ML. Dental enamel formation and implications for Oral health and disease. Physiological Reviews. 2017;**97**(3):939-993

[5] Machiulskiene V, Campus G, Carvalho JC, Dige I, Ekstrand KR, Jablonski-Momeni A, et al. Terminology of dental caries and dental caries management: Consensus report of a workshop organized by ORCA and cariology research group of IADR. Caries Research. 2020;**54**(1):7-14

[6] Robinson C, Shore RC, Brookes SJ, Strafford S, Wood SR, Kirkham J. The chemistry of enamel caries. Critical Reviews in Oral Biology and Medicine. 2000;**11**(4):481-495

[7] Holly FJ, Gray JA. Mechanism for incipient carious lesion growth utilizing a physical model based on diffusion concepts. Archives of Oral Biology. 1968;**13**(3):319-334

[8] Onwubu SC, Mdluli PS, Singh S. Evaluating the buffering and acid-resistant properties of eggshell-titanium dioxide composite against erosive acids. Journal of Applied Biomaterials and Functional Materials. 2019;**17**(1):228

[9] Moreno EC, Zahradnik RT. Chemistry of enamel subsurface demineralization in vitro. Journal of Dental Research. 1974;**53**(2):226-235

[10] Mutahar M, Carpenter G, Bartlett D, German M, Moazzez R. The presence of acquired enamel pellicle changes acid-induced erosion from dissolution to a softening process. Scientific Reports. 2017;**7**(1):10920

[11] Margolis HC, Kwak SY, Yamazaki H. Role of mineralization inhibitors in the regulation of hard tissue biomineralization: Relevance to initial enamel formation and maturation. Frontiers in Physiology. 2014;**5**:339

[12] Brown WE. Physicochemical mechanisms of dental caries. Journal of Dental Research. 1974;**53**(2):204-216

[13] Olek A, Klimek L, Bołtacz-Rzepkowska E. Comparative scanning electron microscope analysis of the enamel of permanent human, bovine and porcine teeth. Journal of Veterinary Science. 2020;**21**(6):e83

[14] De Medeiros RC, Soares JD, De Sousa FB. Natural enamel caries in polarized light microscopy: Differences in histopathological features derived from a qualitative versus a quantitative approach to interpret enamel birefringence. Journal of Microscopy. 2012;**246**(2):177-189

[15] Barbosa de Sousa F, Dias Soares J, Sampaio Vianna S. Natural enamel caries:

A comparative histological study on biochemical volumes. Caries Research. 2013;**47**(3):183-192

[16] Silverstone LM. The surface zone in caries and in caries-like lesions produced in vitro. British Dental Journal. 1968;**125**(4):145-157

[17] Niederberger M, Colfen H. Oriented attachment and mesocrystals: Non-classical crystallization mechanisms based on nanoparticle assembly. Physical Chemistry Chemical Physics. 2006;**8**(28):3271-3287

[18] Dai L, Liu Y, Salameh Z, Khan S, Mao J, Pashley DH, et al. Can caries-affected dentin be completely remineralized by guided tissue remineralization? Dental Hypotheses. 2011;**2**(2):74-82

[19] Boanini E, Torricelli P, Gazzano M, Giardino R, Bigi A. Nanocomposites of hydroxyapatite with aspartic acid and glutamic acid and their interaction with osteoblast-like cells. Biomaterials. 2006;**27**(25):4428-4433

[20] Kawasaki K, Ruben J, Stokroos I, Takagi O, Arends J. The remineralization of EDTA-treated human dentine. Caries Research. 1999;**33**(4):275-280

[21] Xu Z, Neoh KG, Lin CC, Kishen A. Biomimetic deposition of calcium phosphate minerals on the surface of partially demineralized dentine modified with phosphorylated chitosan. Journal of Biomedical Materials Research. Part B, Applied Biomaterials. 2011;**98**(1):150-159

[22] Shellis RP, Finke M, Eisenburger M, Parker DM, Addy M. Relationship between enamel erosion and liquid flow rate. European Journal of Oral Sciences. 2005;**113**(3):232-238

[23] Sivasithamparam K, Young WG, Jirattanasopa V, Priest J, Khan F, Harbrow D, et al. Dental erosion in asthma: A case-control study from south East Queensland. Australian Dental Journal. 2002;**47**(4):298-303

[24] Kargul B, Tanboga I, Ergeneli S, Karakoc F, Dagli E. Inhaler medicament effects on saliva and plaque pH in asthmatic children. The Journal of Clinical Pediatric Dentistry. 1998;**22**(2):137-140

[25] Caufield PW, Griffen AL. Dental caries. An infectious and transmissible disease. Pediatric Clinics of North America. 2000;**47**(5):1001-1019

[26] Douglass JM, Douglass AB, Silk HJ. A practical guide to infant oral health. American Family Physician. 2004;**70**(11):2113-2120

[27] Lussi A, Jaeggi T. Erosion—Diagnosis and risk factors. Clinical Oral Investigations. 2008;**12**(Suppl. 1):S5-S13

[28] Rios D, Honorio HM, Francisconi LF, Magalhaes AC, de Andrade Moreira Machado MA, Buzalaf MA. In situ effect of an erosive challenge on different restorative materials and on enamel adjacent to these materials. Journal of Dentistry. 2008;**36**(2):152-157

[29] Fischer M, Skucha-Nowak M, Chmiela B, Korytkowska-Walach A. Assessment of the potential ability to penetrate into the hard tissues of the root of an experimental preparation with the characteristics of a dental Infiltratant, enriched with an antimicrobial component-preliminary study. Materials (Basel). 2021;**14**(19):53-57

[30] Rocha Gomes Torres C, Borges AB, Torres LM, Gomes IS, de Oliveira RS. Effect of caries infiltration technique and fluoride therapy on the colour

masking of white spot lesions. Journal of Dentistry. 2011;**39**(3):202-207

[31] Silverstone LM. Structure of carious enamel, including the early lesion. Oral Sciences Reviews. 1973;**3**:100-160

[32] Palamara J, Phakey PP, Rachinger WA, Orams HJ. Ultrastructure of the intact surface zone of white spot and brown spot carious lesions in human enamel. Journal of Oral Pathology. 1986;**15**(1):28-35

[33] Darling AI, Mortimer KV, Poole DF, Ollis WD. Molecular sieve behaviour of normal and carious human dental enamel. Archives of Oral Biology. 1961;**5**(3-4):251-273

[34] Paris S, Schwendicke F, Keltsch J, Dorfer C, Meyer-Lueckel H. Masking of white spot lesions by resin infiltration in vitro. Journal of Dentistry. 2013;**41**(Suppl 5):e28-e34

[35] Besnard C, Harper RA, Salvati E, Moxham TEJ, Romano Brandt L, Landini G, et al. Analysis of in vitro demineralised human enamel using multi-scale correlative optical and scanning electron microscopy, and high-resolution synchrotron wide-angle X-ray scattering. Materials & Design. 2021;**206**:109739

[36] Al-Obaidi R, Salehi H, Desoutter A, Bonnet L, Etienne P, Terrer E, et al. Chemical & nano-mechanical Study of artificial human enamel subsurface lesions. Scientific Reports. 2018;**8**(1):4047

[37] Marsh PD. Microbial ecology of dental plaque and its significance in health and disease. Advances in Dental Research. 1994;**8**(2):263-271

[38] Kim MJ, Lee MJ, Kim KM, Yang SY, Seo JY, Choi SH, et al. Enamel demineralization resistance and remineralization by various fluoride-releasing dental restorative materials. Materials (Basel). 2021;**14**(16):223-230

[39] Lussi A, Schlueter N, Rakhmatullina E, Ganss C. Dental erosion—An overview with emphasis on chemical and histopathological aspects. Caries Research. 2011;**45**(Suppl 1):2-12

[40] ten Cate JM. The need for antibacterial approaches to improve caries control. Advances in Dental Research. 2009;**21**(1):8-12

[41] Loesche WJ. The specific plaque hypothesis and the antimicrobial treatment of periodontal disease. Dental Update. 1992;**19**:70

[42] Loesche WJ, Rowan J, Straffon LH, Loos PJ. Association of Streptococcus mutants with human dental decay. Infection and Immunity. 1975;**11**(6):1252-1260

[43] Becker MR, Paster BJ, Leys EJ, Moeschberger ML, Kenyon SG, Galvin JL, et al. Molecular analysis of bacterial species associated with childhood caries. Journal of Clinical Microbiology. 2002;**40**(3):1001-1009

[44] Munson MA, Banerjee A, Watson TF, Wade WG. Molecular analysis of the microflora associated with dental caries. Journal of Clinical Microbiology. 2004;**42**(7):3023-3029

[45] Corby PM, Lyons-Weiler J, Bretz WA, Hart TC, Aas JA, Boumenna T, et al. Microbial risk indicators of early childhood caries. Journal of Clinical Microbiology. 2005;**43**(11):5753-5759

[46] Aas JA, Griffen AL, Dardis SR, Lee AM, Olsen I, Dewhirst FE, et al. Bacteria of dental caries in primary and permanent teeth in children and young

adults. Journal of Clinical Microbiology. 2008;**46**(4):1407-1417

[47] Belda-Ferre P, Alcaraz LD, Cabrera-Rubio R, Romero H, Simon-Soro A, Pignatelli M, et al. The oral metagenome in health and disease. The ISME Journal. 2012;**6**(1): 46-56

[48] Bowden GHW. The microbial ecology of dental caries. Microbial Ecology in Health and Disease. 2009;**12**(3):138-148

[49] Hara AT, Zero DT. The potential of saliva in protecting against dental erosion. Monographs in Oral Science. 2014;**25**:197-205

[50] Navazesh M, Kumar SK. University of Southern California School of D: Measuring salivary flow: Challenges and opportunities. Journal of the American Dental Association (1939). 2008;**139**(Suppl):35S-40S

[51] Aiuchi H, Kitasako Y, Fukuda Y, Nakashima S, Burrow MF, Tagami J. Relationship between quantitative assessments of salivary buffering capacity and ion activity product for hydroxyapatite in relation to cariogenic potential. Australian Dental Journal. 2008;**53**(2):167-171

[52] Miranda-Rius J, Brunet-Llobet L, Lahor-Soler E, Farre M. Salivary secretory disorders, inducing drugs, and clinical management. International Journal of Medical Sciences. 2015;**12**(10):811-824

[53] Javaid MA, Ahmed AS, Durand R, Tran SD. Saliva as a diagnostic tool for oral and systemic diseases. Journal of Oral Biology Craniofacatory Research. 2016;**6**(1):66-75

[54] Aranibar Quiroz EM, Alstad T, Campus G, Birkhed D, Lingstrom P. Relationship between plaque pH and different caries-associated variables in a group of adolescents with varying caries prevalence. Caries Research. 2014;**48**(2):147-153

[55] Aykut-Yetkiner A, Wiegand A, Attin T. The effect of saliva substitutes on enamel erosion in vitro. Journal of Dentistry. 2014;**42**(6):720-725

[56] Reynolds EC. Casein phosphopeptide-amorphous calcium phosphate: The scientific evidence. Advances in Dental Research. 2009;**21**(1):25-29

[57] Cagetti MG, Mastroberardino S, Milia E, Cocco F, Lingstrom P, Campus G. The use of probiotic strains in caries prevention: A systematic review. Nutrients. 2013;**5**(7):2530-2550

[58] Chugh P, Dutt R, Sharma A, Bhagat N, Dhar MS. A critical appraisal of the effects of probiotics on oral health. Journal of Functional Foods. 2020;**70**:103985

[59] Marinho VC, Higgins JP, Logan S, Sheiham A. Topical fluoride (toothpastes, mouthrinses, gels or varnishes) for preventing dental caries in children and adolescents. Cochrane Database of Systematic Reviews. 2003;(4):1-157, CD002782

[60] Benson PE, Parkin N, Dyer F, Millett DT, Germain P. Fluorides for preventing early tooth decay (demineralised lesions) during fixed brace treatment. Cochrane Database of Systematic Reviews. 2019;(11):1-66

[61] Ten Cate JM, Buzalaf MAR. Fluoride mode of action: Once there was an observant dentist. Journal of Dental Research. 2019;**98**(7):725-730

[62] Tasios T, Papageorgiou SN, Papadopoulos MA, Tsapas A, Haidich AB. Prevention of orthodontic enamel demineralization: A systematic review with meta-analyses. Orthodontics & Craniofacial Research. 2019;**22**(4):225-235

[63] Philip N. State of the art enamel remineralization systems: The next frontier in caries management. Caries Research. 2019;**53**(3):284-295

[64] Duckworth RM, Morgan SN. Oral fluoride retention after use of fluoride dentifrices. Caries Research. 1991;**25**(2):123-129

[65] Songsiripradubboon S, Hamba H, Trairatvorakul C, Tagami J. Sodium fluoride mouthrinse used twice daily increased incipient caries lesion remineralization in an in situ model. Journal of Dentistry. 2014;**42**(3):271-278

[66] Wang SP, Ge Y, Zhou XD, Xu HH, Weir MD, Zhang KK, et al. Effect of anti-biofilm glass-ionomer cement on Streptococcus mutans biofilms. International Journal of Oral Science. 2016;**8**(2):76-83

[67] Trairatvorakul C, Techalertpaisarn P, Siwawut S, Ingprapankorn A. Effect of glass ionomer cement and fluoride varnish on the remineralization of artificial proximal caries in situ. The Journal of Clinical Pediatric Dentistry. 2009;**34**(2):131-134

[68] Fernandez CE, Tenuta LMA, Del Bel Cury AA, Nobrega DF, Cury JA. Effect of 5,000 ppm fluoride dentifrice or 1,100 ppm fluoride dentifrice combined with acidulated phosphate fluoride on caries lesion inhibition and repair. Caries Research. 2017;**51**(3):179-187

[69] Silva KG, Pedrini D, Delbem AC, Ferreira L, Cannon M. In situ evaluation of the remineralizing capacity of pit and fissure sealants containing amorphous calcium phosphate and/or fluoride. Acta Odontologica Scandinavica. 2010;**68**(1):11-18

[70] Reynolds EC. Remineralization of enamel subsurface lesions by casein phosphopeptide-stabilized calcium phosphate solutions. Journal of Dental Research. 1997;**76**(9):1587-1595

[71] Cross KJ, Huq NL, Palamara JE, Perich JW, Reynolds EC. Physicochemical characterization of casein phosphopeptide-amorphous calcium phosphate nanocomplexes. The Journal of Biological Chemistry. 2005;**280**(15):15362-15369

[72] Burwell A, Jennings D, Muscle D, Greenspan DC. NovaMin and dentin hypersensitivity—in vitro evidence of efficacy. The Journal of Clinical Dentistry. 2010;**21**(3):66-71

[73] Arifa MK, Ephraim R, Rajamani T. Recent advances in dental hard tissue remineralization: A review of literature. International Journal of Clinical and Pediatrics Dental. 2019;**12**(2):139-144

[74] Sitthisettapong T, Phantumvanit P, Huebner C, Derouen T. Effect of CPP-ACP paste on dental caries in primary teeth: A randomized trial. Journal of Dental Research. 2012;**91**(9):847-852

[75] Prestes L, Souza BM, Comar LP, Salomao PA, Rios D, Magalhaes AC. In situ effect of chewing gum containing CPP-ACP on the mineral precipitation of eroded bovine enamel-a surface hardness analysis. Journal of Dentistry. 2013;**41**(8):747-751

[76] Walker G, Cai F, Shen P, Reynolds C, Ward B, Fone C, et al. Increased remineralization of tooth enamel by milk containing added

casein phosphopeptide-amorphous calcium phosphate. The Journal of Dairy Research. 2006;**73**(1):74-78

[77] Kulal R, Jayanti I, Sambashivaiah S, Bilchodmath S. An In-vitro comparison of Nano hydroxyapatite, Novamin and Proargin desensitizing toothpastes—A SEM study. Journal of Clinical and Diagnostic Research. 2016;**10**(10):ZC51-ZC54

[78] Makinen KK. Sugar alcohols, caries incidence, and remineralization of caries lesions: A literature review. International Journal of Dental. 2010;**2010**:981072

[79] Kusuma Eriwati Y, Putriani D, Geraldine K, Hermansyah H. Fluoride and calcium release from peppermint-flavored fluoride varnish containing dicalcium-phosphate-dihydrate coated with xylitol. Saudi Dental Journal. 2022;**34**(1):68-73

[80] Cummins D. The superior anti-caries efficacy of fluoride toothpaste containing 1.5% arginine. The Journal of Clinical Dentistry. 2016;**27**(2):27-38

[81] Li J, Huang Z, Mei L, Li G, Li H. Anti-caries effect of arginine-containing formulations in vivo: A systematic review and Meta-analysis. Caries Research. 2015;**49**(6):606-617

[82] Cantore R, Petrou I, Lavender S, Santarpia P, Liu Z, Gittins E, et al. In situ clinical effects of new dentifrices containing 1.5% arginine and fluoride on enamel de- and remineralization and plaque metabolism. The Journal of Clinical Dentistry. 2013;**24**:A32-A34

[83] Wolff MS, Schenkel AB. The anticaries efficacy of a 1.5% arginine and fluoride toothpaste. Advances in Dental Research. 2018;**29**(1):93-97

[84] Phan TN, Marquis RE. Triclosan inhibition of membrane enzymes and glycolysis of Streptococcus mutans in suspensions and biofilms. Canadian Journal of Microbiology. 2006;**52**(10):977-983

[85] Riley P, Lamont T. Triclosan/copolymer containing toothpastes for oral health. Cochrane Database of Systematic Reviews. 2013;**2013**(12):CD010514

[86] Silva MF, Giniger MS, Zhang YP, DeVizio W. The effect of a triclosan/copolymer/fluoride liquid dentifrice on interproximal enamel remineralization and fluoride uptake. Journal of the American Dental Association (1939). 2004;**135**(7):1023-1029

[87] Twetman S. Are we ready for caries prevention through bacteriotherapy? Brazilian Oral Research. 2012;**26** (Suppl. 1(SPE1)):64-70

[88] Saha S, Tomaro-Duchesneau C, Rodes L, Malhotra M, Tabrizian M, Prakash S. Investigation of probiotic bacteria as dental caries and periodontal disease biotherapeutics. Benefeciary Microbes. 2014;**5**(4):447-460

[89] Cildir SK, Germec D, Sandalli N, Ozdemir FI, Arun T, Twetman S, et al. Reduction of salivary mutans streptococci in orthodontic patients during daily consumption of yoghurt containing probiotic bacteria. European Journal of Orthodontics. 2009;**31**(4):407-411

[90] Epasinghe DJ, Kwan S, Chu D, Lei MM, Burrow MF, Yiu CKY. Synergistic effects of proanthocyanidin, tri-calcium phosphate and fluoride on artificial root caries and dentine collagen. Materials Science & Engineering. C, Materials for Biological Applications. 2017;**73**:293-299

[91] Bhalodia NR, Shukla VJ. Antibacterial and antifungal activities

from leaf extracts of Cassia fistula l.: An ethnomedicinal plant. Journal of Advanced Pharmaceutical Technology & Research. 2011;**2**(2):104-109

[92] Khalid GS, Hamrah MH, Ghafary ES, Hosseini S, Almasi F. Antibacterial and antimicrobial effects of Xanthorrhizol in the prevention of dental caries: A systematic review. Drug Design, Development and Therapy. 2021;**15**:1149-1156

[93] Celik ZC, Yavlal GO, Yanikoglu F, Kargul B, Tagtekin D, Stookey GK, et al. Do ginger extract, natural honey and bitter chocolate remineralize enamel surface as fluoride toothpastes? An In-vitro study. Nigerian Journal of Clinical Practice. 2021;**24**(9):1283-1288

[94] Bilgin Gocmen G, Yanikoglu F, Tagtekin D, Stookey GK, Schemehorn BR, Hayran O. Effectiveness of some herbals on initial enamel caries lesion. Asian Pacific Journal of Tropical Biomedicine. 2016;**6**(10):846-850

Chapter 3

The Influence of Salivary pH on the Prevalence of Dental Caries

Laura-Cristina Rusu, Alexandra Roi, Ciprian-Ioan Roi, Codruta Victoria Tigmeanu and Lavinia Cosmina Ardelean

Abstract

Dental caries is the most prevalent chronic oral disease, influencing the oral and systemic health of the individuals, being the result of the interaction of multiple factors, such as microbial agents, the oral environment, the salivary pH, and the host response. The main process that occurs in dental caries is the demineralization of the tooth enamel, process that is directly influenced by the salivary pH, exposing the dental structures to the action of pathological agents. The role of saliva in the etiology of dental caries is a major one, by influencing the homeostasis through the altering of its buffer capacity. The properties of saliva are influenced either by local pathogens or through a general mechanism with direct implications upon the salivary components. The alteration of the salivary pH, flow rate, and composition will further have repercussions upon the cariogenic activity, through a change of its physiochemical properties. Nevertheless, the salivary pH is strongly linked to the incidence of dental caries, any persistent imbalance due to various causes can be assessed as an indicator of the oral health status.

Keywords: dental caries, salivary pH, oral pathology, oral health, dentistry, buffer capacity

1. Introduction

Dental caries is considered one of the most common chronic diseases affecting the global population [1]. An important aspect associated to dental caries is the potential serious consequences upon the general health of the individuals [2]. Previous studies stated the fact that oral bacteria can spread and determine various systemic health implications, being responsible for secondary infections of different organs [2]. Multiple research studies discuss the involvement of persistent oral bacteria, due to an inadequate oral hygiene, specific dental procedures or periodontitis in the initiation of endocarditis [3]. The oral environment can be influenced, as well, by the general health status and treatments with a direct impact upon the oral microbiota balance, the salivary flow, and pH. A high interest has been shown in identifying the composition, properties, and implications of the oral microbiome and its consequences upon the salivary pH, oral pathologies, and systemic diseases. The prevalence of dental caries is still characterized by high values despite the prevention measures applied worldwide. Its incidence continues to increase dramatically once the risk habits prevalence in the developing countries changes. However, it has been reported that a small percentage of young adults can still be characterized as being caries-free. Unfortunately, the efforts to identify risk populations by using a screening method had no significant result [4].

The etiology and the pathogenesis of dental caries are being considered complex multifactorial processes [5]. An important role is assigned to saliva, its rate and composition being most important in the initiation and progression of the cariogenic process. Being the body fluid, which is in permanent contact with the teeth and soft oral tissues, it is held responsible for their integrity and for the permanent remineralization of the dental structures, as well. The quantity of the salivary flow, the characteristics of saliva, and its buffer capacity are involved in maintaining a proper balance of the oral environment. Any alterations of these characteristics can influence the demineralization process and are consequently responsible for the development of caries. The salivary components may have a substantial implication in the reduction of the risk factors involved in dental caries incidence [5].

The factors associated with occurrence of dental caries are the host (the presence of teeth and saliva), the oral microbiome (the bacterial population), and the dietary habits (based on carbohydrates). Basically, all these factors contribute and conduct to the development of the disease. Caries is characterized by a progressive evolution, being reversible in early stages, and suggesting that the abovementioned factors must have a cumulative action for a certain period of time. Dental caries is the result of the interaction between the oral microbiome accumulated on teeth's surface (dental plaque) with the fermentable sugars form the diet, with consequences upon the buffering capacity of the saliva, lowering its pH, and weakening the normal remineralization process [6].

The demineralization and remineralization cycles of the enamel, under the action of the cariogenic bacteria from the dental plaque, are quite frequent mechanisms that occur in the oral cavity, episodically. Enamel has a unique structure, without any organic components that could contribute to its repair or defense against a potential cariogenic attempt. In the early stages of the demineralization process, the action of saliva combined with the mechanical removal of the dental plaque and application of topic fluorides may stop and reverse the process.

An accurate evaluation of the dental caries risk should take in consideration the implication of saliva in the process. The use of a salivary test in the assessment of the individual risk may have an impact upon the prevention strategies, screening, and early diagnosis of dental caries, making a difference in the incidence statistics of dental caries [6].

2. Saliva and its functions

The oral cavity and the teeth are permanently exposed to the action of saliva [7]. The oral fluid is the result of the secretion of multiple salivary glands: the parotid, submandibular, sublingual, and the minor salivary glands localized in multiple areas of the oral mucosa. Free epithelial cells, bacteria, crevicular fluid, inflammatory cells, and food particles are among the components of saliva. The implications of saliva and its functions contribute to the maintenance of the oral health [8]. One of its main roles is hydrating and lubrication of the surrounding tissues. The submandibular, parotid, sublingual, and minor salivary glands contribute with 60, 25, 8, and

7%, respectively, to the whole saliva amount, when in unstimulated state. In case of salivary flow stimulation, their secretion increases with at least 10% [9]. The salivary flow varies from 0.3 ml/min up to 1.5–2.0 ml/min, depending of the state: stimulation period or rest. There are circadian variations involved, as well, during the day 0.5 liter of saliva is secreted, compared with night when the flow rate is highly decreased [9].

Saliva and its actions are dependent on its quantity and quality. Being in permanent contact with the oral tissues, it has influence on actions such as speaking, swallowing, and eating, protecting the mucosa and the surface of the teeth. The protective role of the saliva is supported by a proper viscosity, flow rate, balanced composition, pH, and buffer function [10]. Any alterations of these characteristics may result in developing oral pathologies such as dental caries (**Figure 1**).

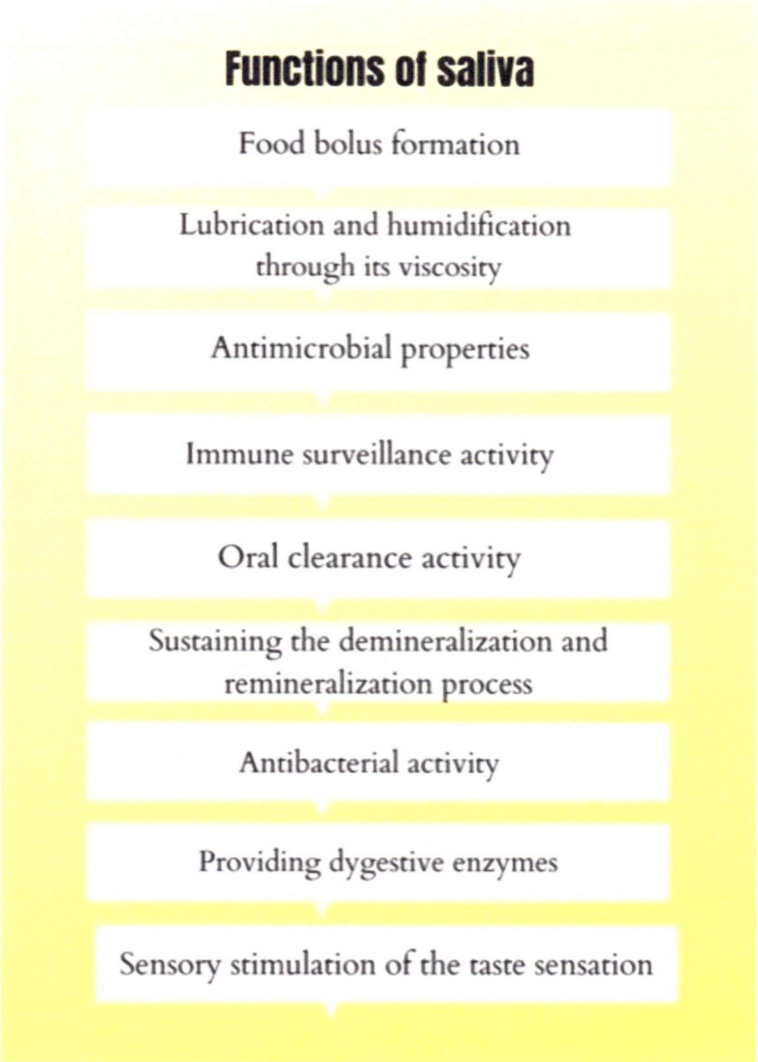

Figure 1.
Roles and functions of the saliva.

To date, research has focused on identifying the relationship between the characteristics of saliva and the incidence of dental caries. Several studies reported that there was a connection between the viscosity of saliva and the development of dental caries [8]. The high cariogenic activity due to the alteration of the salivary characteristics could be explained by a reduced flow rate, a decreased clearance and buffer capacity, and a high glucose concentration. It has been shown that the salivary flow rate was significantly lower in individuals with active caries compared with caries-free ones [11]. The buffer capacity and the pH values have direct consequences upon the salivary flow rate and viscosity [10].

The composition and flow rate of saliva vary in relation with different factors, such as stimulation or rest periods [10]. In the rest periods, the salivary flow rate represents ¼ out of the total stimulated flow potential. During the stimulated flow, the composition and pH of the saliva change, a more serious saliva consistency facilitates the digestive process and increases the clearance function [12]. The immune surveillance role of the saliva is due to immunoglobulins, secreted by the plasma cells of the lymphoid tissue belonging to the major salivary glands. The epithelial cells localized in the salivary acini produce proteins with a protective role against bacteria and viruses.

Because of its complex composition, saliva has multiple actions in the oral environment. In vitro studies, focused on the interaction between the cariogenic microorganisms in the dental plaque and the salivary proteins, suggest that interleukins, lysozyme, mucins, and lactotransferrin contribute to the cell aggregation, inhibition action, and adherence of the bacteria, suggesting that the salivary proteins may have a diagnostic potential, allowing the development of personalized treatments [13, 14].

Dental caries is represented by a localized demineralization with progressive loss of the tooth components. The healthy oral environment is in symbiosis with the oral microbiome, in case of a neutral pH value. The bacteria from the oral biofilm are responsible for metabolizing the carbohydrates and producing permanent organic acid products, which are able to lower the pH, with effects upon the tooth

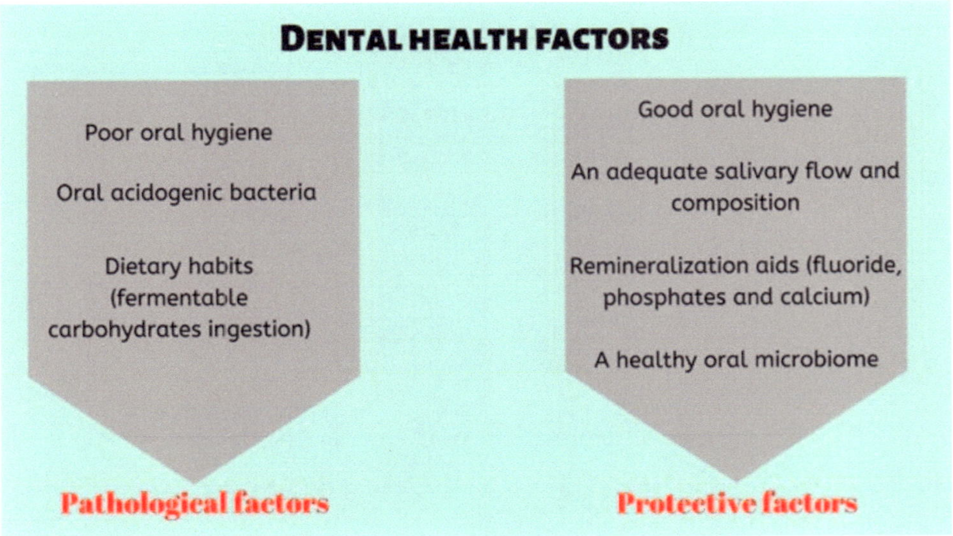

Figure 2.
The contribution of the pathological and protective factors.

composition and biofilm [15]. A long-time persistence of a lower pH value influences the bacterial population of the biofilm, producing a shift in the oral microbiome and promoting the acidogenic bacteria [16]. These changes will eventually have repercussions upon the oral environment by the acidification process. A low pH value will result in the extraction of phosphate and calcium from the tooth structures, in order to attempt to equilibrate the acid environment, determining their demineralization. These types of actions take place several times per day and are being influenced by numerous other mechanisms and factors such as oral hygiene, diet, oral microbiome diversity, genetics, dental anatomy, biofilm, salivary flow, buffer capacity, and composition (**Figure 2**).

Saliva has an important role in maintaining a healthy oral environment and proper digestion, and its alterations can be the cause of multiple diseases, including dental caries.

3. Salivary pH and buffer capacity

The buffer capacity of saliva plays an important role in mediating the relationship between the tooth surface and the biofilm, normally exhibiting a protective role against the development of dental caries [17]. This specific characteristic of saliva is represented by the concentration of the bicarbonate ion. The buffer capacity may be quantified and assessed, in case of active-caries individuals, by a titration method, from salivary samples. The implications of the buffer action rely on reducing the acid formation in the dental biofilm. In case of a pathogenic action, the neutralization of an acidic pH environment, and shifting it into a neutral one, has proven to be quite difficult [18].

The composition of saliva has an important contribution in maintaining and increasing the value of the pH biofilm. Among its main constituents, which efficiently determine the pH to increase are sialin (that contains arginine and lysine) and urea. Further hydrolyzation of each of these molecules results in releasing ammonia, with a direct contribution in increasing the pH.

In order to maintain the oral health and the integrity of the tooth surface, the pH value should be kept around the value of 6.7. The ion concentration and activity are responsible for demineralization and remineralization processes through the solubility of hydroxyapatite [19]. A decreased and critical pH value is considered at a value of/under 5.5.

The pH value is directly related to the concentration of the phosphate and calcium ions. Salivary flow and its variations have consequences upon the pH value, by exhibiting different concentrations of calcium and phosphate. It has been reported that the pH value can be increased by one unit only through stimulating the salivary flow rate. Differences between the unstimulated and stimulated saliva have been identified, as the unstimulated saliva has a lower pH value compared with the stimulated one, due to its higher concentration in phosphate [20]. The critical pH value presents individual variations, as the salivary concentrations of calcium and phosphate vary from one person to another. It should also be mentioned that the critical pH fluctuations are dependent on multiple factors [21].

Saliva has three buffering systems, which are represented by phosphate, bicarbonate, and protein systems. The major system being considered is the acid/bicarbonate one, present in the stimulated salivary secretion. Its action starts with food intake, by decreasing the pH value and increasing the concentration of bicarbonate. The phosphate buffer system and its effectiveness are dependent on the salivary concentration of the phosphate ion and have been reported to have a moderate action in case of unstimulated saliva [22]. The salivary proteins represent another buffer system, through their action of absorbing and releasing protons. Their action may result in increasing the saliva viscosity when the pH value is low, protecting the tooth structure from acid production, by exhibiting a physical barrier [20].

The pH value during rest periods has been reported to have the ability to predict the caries status of the patient and outline the buffering capacity of the saliva. Patients with resting salivary pH value of approximately 7.0 have been reported to have a lower caries activity compared with those with pH values of 5.5, who exhibited a high caries incidence. In individuals with pH values between 5.5 and 7.0, the caries incidence was less severe. A lower value of a resting pH suggests a lower pH value when exposed to carbohydrates, with a prolonged maintenance of this lower value, until returning to the resting pH [8]. These facts suggest that the changes during a lower pH value result in exposing the tooth structure to an acidic environment, for a longer period of time, without the possibility of neutralizing it.

The presence of dental caries influences the carbohydrate clearance, resulting in a prolonged contact with the dental plaque and a continuous decrease of the salivary pH value [11]. The presence of dental caries and alteration of the oral environment promote the production of acid, supplementary bacterial adhesion, and low salivary clearance activity. A previous published study concluded that the salivary flow rate, the buffer capacity, and pH value were decreased in active-caries children compared with the caries-free group [23].

The implication of the salivary pH in the multiplication and survival of oral microorganisms is an important aspect in the etiology of dental caries. In case of a low pH, the acidophilic microorganisms will multiply, considerably increasing the caries risk [24]. A high incidence of dental caries, dysphagia, and other oral pathologies has been linked to a decreased salivary flow, clearance, and buffer capacity. Special attention should be paid to the patients with decreased saliva secretion, with repercussions upon the oral mucosa, upon the viscosity and buffer capacity, favoring the development of opportunistic infections and increasing the risk of dental caries [25].

4. PH variations and dental caries risk in systemic conditions

The oral cavity and the salivary composition and characteristics may be defined as the mirror of the general health status. Saliva represents the first body fluid, which comes in contact with multiple pathogens, being responsible for their neutralization, and for the homeostasis of the oral environment. Recent studies have revealed the importance of assessing the levels of salivary antioxidants and reactive oxygen species, which have a high implication in the incidence of dental caries.

A clinical study conducted on children diagnosed with iron deficiency anemia revealed its impact upon the salivary pH value and buffer capacity. By collecting unstimulated saliva and serum samples from the patients, before and after treatment, the salivary buffer capacity and pH values have been quantified. The serum ferritin levels were measured, in order to outline their role as dental caries and iron deficiency anemia biomarkers. The results showed that 3 months after treatment, the buffering capacity and the salivary pH have increased, suggesting a direct implication of the iron deficiency anemia in altering the salivary functions with secondary implications in the cariogenic activity [26].

The salivary dysfunction related to primary Sjögren's syndrome may be the cause of multiple oral manifestations. The results of several studies discuss the fact that patients diagnosed with primary Sjögren's syndrome have a high incidence of dental caries, exhibiting mostly cervical carious lesions, despite an acceptable oral hygiene status [27]. Several salivary factors that have been encountered in primary Sjögren's syndrome patients have been linked to the high incidence of caries. The main problem related to this pathology is the influence upon the saliva formation, patients experiencing a decreased salivary flow rate, and an alteration in the salivary composition, due to the presence of focal lymphocytic infiltrate in the salivary glands. Pedersen et al. [28] conducted a study that aimed to identify and evaluate the salivary flow and composition and the incidence of dental caries in patients diagnosed with primary Sjögren's syndrome. The results showed that the included patients exhibited a decreased salivary flow rate, and the pH and bicarbonate concentration of the parotid gland's saliva were significantly decreased compared with the control group. Although patients had accurate oral hygiene habits and reported using dental floss and fluoride toothpaste, the caries incidence and gingival index were high. These patients also had a higher number of acidophilic, cariogenic bacteria in the dental plaque compared with the control group, and a relationship between the decreased salivary flow and the high incidence of Lactobacillus has been observed. Among all the oral manifestations, oral dryness and a reduced salivary flow rate were the main accuses of the patients [29].

A decreased salivary flow has been reported in diabetic patients, the incidence of type I diabetes among young patients may have repercussions on the oral health, especially teeth integrity. The association between dental caries and diabetes has been one of the most researched subjects. As type I diabetes is associated with the critical years of dental eruption, the attention in identifying its potential implication on the dental status has been considered a necessity. Studies have reported a high incidence of dental caries, dry mouth (xerostomia), and gingival inflammation in young patients diagnosed with type I diabetes compared with healthy ones. One of the main causes that could explain this outcome, besides a poor oral hygiene, could be the decreased salivary flow rate and alteration of the composition of saliva. Elevated glucose concentration has been identified in the saliva, sustaining an acidogenic oral environment and the colonization of bacteria. All these changes in the flow rate, salivary composition, and an inadequate oral hygiene influence the incidence of dental caries [29]. Studies including patients with type I diabetes showed that the salivary flow and pH value were significantly reduced compared with the control group, the prevalence and severity of dental caries in type I diabetes being a high one [29].

High incidence of dental caries, mucositis, and inflammation has been identified in acute lymphoblastic leukemia. The main changes are related to the compromised immune system, influencing the oral environment as well. Hegde et al. [30] conducted a study focusing on the implication of acute lymphoblastic leukemia on the oral health and dental status. They aimed to identify the direct action of the disease, as well as the influence of chemotherapy on the salivary flow and dental caries incidence. The study included patients divided into four groups (without chemotherapy, at the beginning of chemotherapy treatment, after 4 weeks of chemotherapy, and a control group). The results showed that all three groups with acute lymphoblastic leukemia experienced a low salivary flow rate and pH values compared with the control group. The antioxidant salivary levels were increased in the first two groups and decreased in the third group of leukemia patients. Poor oral hygiene and gingival inflammation were reported in all leukemia patients, and the incidence of dental caries was a high one. The influence of chemotherapy on the salivary flow through the hypoplasia of the salivary glands is a common consequence of this treatment. Another cause for the poor dental health status, besides the abovementioned salivary changes, could be the discomfort caused by the inflammation of the oral mucosa that reduces the possibility of maintaining a proper oral hygiene [30].

The role of saliva in the diagnosis of multiple diseases through its composition and actions is currently accepted. The salivary secretion is controlled by a reflex arc influenced by multiple actions. For the salivary flow and composition, the parasympathetic and sympathetic systems are responsible. Multiple studies were conducted in identifying the stress-related consequence upon the saliva [31]. Results show an increase in the acidity levels of saliva in case of anxiety and a decrease of the salivary flow and pH value with consequences upon the tooth structure [31]. Said et al. [32] conducted a study, which aimed to identify the relationship between the anxiety levels and the changes encountered in the saliva. The results outline the existence of a low pH value in the study group, compared with the control group, revealing a higher prevalence among males with a low anxiety level. These alterations could be a further explanation for the prevalence of dental caries among these patients.

Systemic health plays an important role in maintaining an adequate oral environment. Changes specific to various diseases can directly influence the salivary production, composition, and functions, with influence on the prevalence of dental caries. Over the past years, research has opened a new path that includes the use of saliva for screening, diagnosis, and monitoring of multiple pathologies.

5. Conclusions

Among the numerous factors linked to the incidence of dental caries, the oral microorganisms and saliva are of most importance. The role of saliva cannot be underestimated, its composition revealing important information regarding the involvement of systemic and oral conditions. Research has focused on outlining the importance of the salivary functions and characteristics in the development of dental caries. Connections between the pH values and the prevalence of caries have been pointed out, the influence of local and general factors, as well as the impact of pH variations upon the tooth structure. An acidogenic oral environment results in an imbalanced demineralization and remineralization process, with a multiplying community of acidophilic bacteria. The key in the management of dental caries is addressing the causative factors, both general and local, and obtaining a neutral oral pH.

Conflict of interest

The authors declare no conflict of interest.

Author details

Laura-Cristina Rusu[1], Alexandra Roi[1], Ciprian-Ioan Roi[2], Codruta Victoria Tigmeanu[3] and Lavinia Cosmina Ardelean[3]*

1 Department of Oral Pathology, Multidisciplinary Center for Research, Evaluation, Diagnosis and Therapies in Oral Medicine, "Victor Babes" University of Medicine and Pharmacy, Timisoara, Romania

2 Department of Anaesthesiology and Oral Surgery, Multidisciplinary Center for Research, Evaluation, Diagnosis and Therapies in Oral Medicine, "Victor Babes" University of Medicine and Pharmacy, Timisoara, Romania

3 Department of Technology of Materials and Devices in Dental Medicine, Multidisciplinary Center for Research, Evaluation, Diagnosis and Therapies in Oral Medicine, "Victor Babeş," University of Medicine and Pharmacy, Timisoara, Romania

*Address all correspondence to: lavinia_ardelean@umft.ro

References

[1] Frencken JE, Sharma P, Stenhouse L, Green D, Laverty D, Dietrich T. Global epidemiology of dental caries and severe periodontitis - a comprehensive review. Journal of Clinical Periodontology. 2017;**44**(Suppl. 18):S94e105

[2] Kim JK, Baker LA, Davarian S, Crimmins E. Oral health problems and mortality. Journal of Dental Science. 2013;**8**:115-120. DOI: 10.1016/j.jds.2012.12.011

[3] Kriebel K, Hieke C, Muller-Hilke B, Nakata M, Kreikemeyer B. Oral biofilms from symbiotic to pathogenic interactions and associated disease-connection of periodontitis and rheumatic arthritis by peptidylarginine deiminase. Frontiers in Microbiology. 2018;**9**:53

[4] Anderson MH. Current concepts of dental caries and its prevention. Operative Dentistry Supplement. 2001;**6**:11-18

[5] Vellore G, Arzreanne AR. Saliva as a diagnostic tool for assessment of dental caries. Archives of Orofacial Sciences. 2006;**1**:57-59

[6] Jepsen S, Blanco J, Buchalla W, Carvalho JC, Dietrich T, Dörfer C, et al. Prevention and control of dental caries and periodontal diseases at individual andpopulation level: Consensus report of group 3 of joint EFP/ORCA workshop on the boundaries between caries and periodontal diseases. Journal of Clinical Periodontology. 2017;**44**(Suppl. 44):S85-S93. DOI: 10.1111/jcpe.12687

[7] Sreebny LM. Saliva in health and disease: An appraisal and update. International Dental Journal. 2000;**50**:140-161

[8] Hicks J, Garcia-Godoy F, Flaitz C. Biological factors in dental caries: Role of saliva and dental plaque in the dynamic process of demineralization and remineralization (part 1). Journal of Clinical Pediatric Dentistry. 2004;**28**:47-52

[9] Khan GJ, Javed M, Ishaq M. Effect of smoking on salivary flow rate. International Journal of Molecular Sciences. 2010;**8**:221-225

[10] Lagerlöf F, Oliveby A. Caries-protective factors in saliva. Advances in Dental Research. 1994;**8**:229-238. DOI: 10.1177/08959374940080021601

[11] Aminabadi NA, Najafpour E, Rohani ZR, Deljavan AS, Ghojazadeh M, Jamali Z. Linear reciprocal interaction between dental caries and salivary characteristics. Journal of Oral Science. 2013;**55**:337-342

[12] Schenkels LCPM, Veerman ECI, Amerongen AVN. Biochemical composition of human saliva in relation to other mucosal fluids. Critical Reviews in Oral Biology & Medicine. 1995;**6**:161-175

[13] Cogulu D, Onay H, Ozdemir Y, Aslan I, G, Ozkinay F, Kutukculer N, Eronat C. Associations of interleukin (IL)-1β, IL-1 receptor antagonist, and IL-10 with dental caries. Journal of Oral Science. 2015;**57**:31-36. DOI: 10.2334/josnusd.57.31

[14] Andrade FB, Oliveira JC, Yoshie MT, Guimarães BM, Gonçalves RB, Schwarcz WD. Antimicrobial activity and synergism of lactoferrin and lysozyme against cariogenic microorganisms. Brazilian Dental Journal. 2014;**25**:165-169. DOI: 10.1590/0103-6440201302257

[15] Takahashi N, Nyvad B. The role of bacteria in the caries process: Ecological perspectives. Journal of Dental Research. 2011;**90**:294-303

[16] Ferjeskov O, Nyvad B, Kidd E. Dental Caries: The Disease and its Clinical Management. 3rd ed. Oxford: Wiley-Blackwell; 2015 480p

[17] Xiao J, Klein MI, Falsetta ML, Lu B, Delahunty CM, Yates JR III, et al. The exopolysaccharide matrix modulates the interaction between 3D architecture and virulence of a mixed-species oral biofilm. PLoS Pathogens. 2012;**8**:e1002623. DOI: 10.1371/journal.ppat.1002623

[18] Koo H, Falsetta ML, Klein MI. The exopolysaccharide matrix: A virulence determinant of cariogenic biofilm. Journal of Dental Research. 2013;**92**:1065-1073

[19] Aframian DJ, Davidowitz T, Benoliel R. The distribution of oral mucosal pH values in healthy saliva secretors. Oral Disease. 2006;**12**:420-423

[20] Ramezani J, Khaligh MR, Ansari G, Yazdani Y, Mohammadi S. Association of salivary physicochemical characteristics and peptide levels with dental caries in children. Journal of Indian Society of Pedodontics and Preventive Dentistry. 2021;**39**:189-195

[21] Dawes C. What is the critical pH and why does a tooth dissolve in acid? Journal of Canadian Dental Association. 2003;**69**:722-724

[22] Bardow A, Moe D, Nyvad B, Nauntofte B. The buffer capacity and buffer systems of human whole saliva measured without loss of CO2. Archives of Oral Biology. 2000;**45**:1-2

[23] Gandhy M, Damle SG. Relation of salivary inorganic phosphorus and alkaline phosphatase to the dental caries status in children. Journal of Indian Society of Pedodontics and Preventive Dentistry. 2003;**21**:135-138

[24] Jeong SJ, Apostolska S, Jankulovska M, Angelova D, Nares S, Yoon MS, et al. Dental caries risk can be predicted by simply measuring the pH and buffering capacity of saliva. Journal of Dental Hygiene Science. 2006;**6**:159-162

[25] Mojabi KB, Esfahani M, Hashemi HJ. Evaluation of unstimulated salivary flow rate and oral symptoms in menopausal women. Journal of Dentistry Tehran. 2007;**4**:103-106

[26] Mahantesha T, Reddy KP, Ellore VPK, Ramagoni NK, Iitagi V, Anitha KS. Evaluation and association of iron deficiency anemia with salivary pH and buffering capacity in children aged 6-12 years. National Journal of Physiology, Pharmacy and Pharmacology. 1970;**4**:229-229

[27] Pedersen AM, Nauntofte B. Primary Sjögren's syndrome: Oral aspects on pathogenesis, diagnostic criteria, clinical features and approaches for therapy. Expert Opinion on Pharmacotherapy. 2001;**2**:1415-1436

[28] Pedersen AML, Bardow A, Nauntofte B. Salivary changes and dental caries as potential oral markers of autoimmune salivary gland dysfunction in primary Sjögren's syndrome. BMC Clinical Pathology. 2005;**5**:1-13

[29] Rai K, Hegde A, Kamath A, Shetty S. Dental caries and salivary alterations in type I diabetes. Journal of Clinical Pediatric Dentistry. 2011;**36**:181-184

[30] Hegde AM, Joshi S, Rai K, Shetty S. Evaluation of oral hygiene status, salivary characteristics and

dental caries experience in acute lymphoblastic leukemic (ALL) children. Journal of Clinical Pediatric Dentistry. 2011;**35**:319-323

[31] Yaribeygi H, Panahi Y, Sahraei H, Johnston TP, Sahebkar A. The impact of stress on body function: A review. EXCLI Journal. 2017;**16**:1057-1072

[32] Said OB, Razumova S, Velichko E, Tikhonova S, Barakat H. Evaluation of the changes of salivary pH among dental students depending on their anxiety level. European Journal of Dentistry. 2020;**14**:605-612

Chapter 4

Diet and Nutrition and Their Relationship with Early Childhood Dental Caries

Luanna Gonçalves Ferreira,
Giuliana de Campos Chaves Lamarque
and Francisco Wanderley Garcia Paula-Silva

Abstract

Early consumption of foods containing sugar is increasing and one of the consequences of this exposure is caries in early childhood, that is, in children under 6 years of age. Early consumption results in the child's taste and food choice throughout life, maintaining cariogenic dietary patterns. It is important to emphasize that most eating behaviors occur due to family influence. Therefore, an approach in dental prenatal care and consultations until the first year of age, allows the establishment of eating habits and oral hygiene, as well as guidelines and instructions for the adoption of certain measures that contribute to the health of pregnant women and babies. Based on the present study, we conclude the importance of establishing the relationship between the dentist and the pregnant woman, since early educational actions act directly on health in the gestational period and the child's growth. The early consumption of sugar is correlated with the occurrence of caries in early childhood due to family habits. Therefore, it becomes relevant instructions that help in maintaining healthy nutritional habits and correct oral hygiene practices, since focusing on educational actions increases the chances of healthy gestational and infant development.

Keywords: early childhood dental caries, diet, dysbiosis, sugar, oral health education

1. Introduction

In recent decades with the global nutritional transition, there has been an increase in the consumption of sugary drinks and processed foods rich in carbohydrates by children [1]. Cariogenic bacteria ferment sugar and carbohydrates from the diet, promoting a decrease in oral pH for values that favor demineralization and creating a favorable ecological environment for the survival of cariogenic microorganisms [2]. The acids produced by the fermentation of sugar by the bacteria that make up the biofilm cause an imbalance between demineralization and remineralization, leading to the loss of minerals in the dental hard tissues, the important sign being white spot lesions followed by cavitation of a caries lesion [3].

It is noteworthy that the consumption of foods and beverages with sugar in early life has been associated with an increased risk of overweight, obesity, and non-communicable diseases, such as cardiovascular diseases, type 2 diabetes, and dental caries [4, 5]. The main oral disease in children is dental caries, often related to the consumption of free sugars contained in food or supplemented [6]. In addition, approximately 30% of children are born with development defects in tooth enamel, which favors the risk of caries in these children [7].

Dental caries is a dynamic and multifactorial disease mediated by biofilm, modulated by diet, and non-transmissible, determined by biological, behavioral, psychosocial, and environmental factors of caries [8, 9]. It is one of the most prevalent preventable diseases, being reported in more than 90% of children between 3 and 5 years in some countries [10].

Caries in early childhood are characterized by the presence of one or more cavities in one or more deciduous teeth in children under 6 years [11]. The International Association of Paediatric Dentistry (IAPD) recommends avoiding the ingestion of sugar by children under two years [12]. However, studies report large consumption of foods and beverages with sugar by children, before completing the first year of life [13, 14]. One of the main preventive strategies for the management of caries in early childhood is to provide caregivers with instructions on a balanced diet and effective strategies to prevent the accumulation of biofilm on the tooth surface [12].

2. Overview

The early and increasing consumption of sugar-containing foods and beverages in different communities of the world and the understanding of the role of sugar as a common risk factor for different adverse health outcomes indicate the need for urgent measures [13, 15, 16]. Caries in early childhood are the first clinically important result stemming from the early introduction of sugar and can affect children before they even complete the first year of life [12]. It is also essential to conduct an early dental consultation for follow-up and counseling before teeth eruption, in which parents and caregivers have the opportunity to receive information about oral health, which can increase awareness about appropriate oral hygiene behaviors and practices [17].

3. Diet and dental caries

The oral microbiota has a symbiotic relationship with the host, where it provides a favorable habitat for the growth of several microorganisms and in return, these microorganisms provide several benefits, such as the development of the immune system [18]. Its biological function and architecture are determined by the composition and properties of saliva and, more importantly, by the dominant nutritional source in the child's diet [19]. The mineralized surface of the teeth allows the colonization of several microorganisms, including *Streptococcus mutans and Streptococcus sobrinus*, which are acid-producing cariogenic bacteria [20].

Therefore, in the presence of fermentable carbohydrates, the acid produced by these bacteria begins to demineralize the surface enamel or the outermost layer of the teeth, initiating the caries lesion [20]. With this, biofilm alone is not able to provoke dental caries, but exposure to dietary sugars and the individual's ability to overcome cariogenic challenges are determining factors for its occurrence [21].

Therefore, caries is a diet-related disease [22]. Other factors that contribute to the cause of dental caries are salivary flow rate, buffering capacity, i.e., saliva's ability to neutralize acids and maintain its pH, and the availability of some enzymes and protective molecules in saliva [11]. In the early stages of the disease, before cavitation, the progression of carious injury can be interrupted and even reversed, mainly by reducing the consumption of free sugar and encouraging behavioral changes that favor remineralization processes [23].

The risk of caries attributable to dietary factors is influenced by both food choices and eating behaviors. Three factors interact to determine the risk of caries associated with an individual's diet: sugar intake, frequency of consumption, and duration of the feeding [22]. Thus, the early supply of sweetened foods and beverages can have significant dental consequences, potentially laying the foundations for future cariogenic dietary patterns or dysbiosis in the oral cavity [15].

In relation to sugar intake, eating patterns in childhood, characterized by a greater number of highly sweetened foods and beverages in the first year of age, are strongly associated with the incidence of childhood caries in subsequent years [15]. The purchase of sugary foods by the family is a reflection of family consumption, not necessarily of the child. However, considering that young children quickly develop dietary patterns similar to those of their families, it is plausible that purchases interfered with sugar intake, reflected in the association with dental caries [24].

Moreover, the ubiquitous availability of sugary foods and beverages in contemporary household environments is associated with a decrease in balanced food meals, thus, the frequency of consumption becomes prolonged, increasing the opportunity for fermentation of carbohydrates in the oral cavity and subsequent risk of caries [22].

Therefore, the first years of life can represent a key opportunity for intervention, helping to establish a trajectory of low sugar content and low caries content throughout life, contrary to a trajectory intertwined between caries and sugar intake throughout life [25, 26].

4. Caries in early childhood

Caries in early childhood is defined as dental caries in children under 6 years of age, in which nutritional risk factors, such as bottle feeding and frequent consumption of sugary drinks and carbohydrate-rich snacks, as well as inadequate tooth brushing and limited access to fluoride and dental care, contribute to its occurrence [1, 12, 27, 28].

In addition to the consumption of fermentable carbohydrates with high frequency by children, other indicators of risk of caries in early childhood are if the mother or caregiver has active caries lesions, the situation and socioeconomic status of the family [29]. Epidemiological data from a 2011–2012 United States survey indicate that caries in early childhood remains highly prevalent in poor and almost poor preschool children [30]. The experience of caries in the deciduous dentition is one of the strongest predictors of caries experience in permanent dentition [31].

As a result, the American Academy of Pediatric Dentistry (AAPD) encourages professionals to adapt and instruct home preventive measures that provide evidence-based prevention of caries in early childhood, such as: establishing contact with a dentist within 6 months after the eruption of the first tooth and at the latest at 12 months of age to perform caries risk assessment, parents' education and anticipatory guidance [32]. In addition, it is also necessary to modify diets to avoid frequent consumption of liquids and/or solid foods containing sugar [33]. The implementation of oral hygiene measures must be carried out at the time of the eruption of the first deciduous tooth [32].

5. Prevention of dental caries

Strategies to prevent caries in early childhood should begin with the education of the parents and/or caregivers during the prenatal period and progress through the perinatal period [28]. The family approach can be an effective solution, where families receive oral health education to ensure the early adoption of healthy behaviors, such as correct tooth brushing with toothpaste containing at least 1,100 ppm of fluoride and flossing, adoption of appropriate eating practices, reduction of the amount and frequency of sugar consumption and search for dental care before the baby's first tooth eruption [34, 35]. The International Association of Pediatric Dentistry (IAPD) recommends that this toothbrushing be performed at least twice a day with fluoride toothpaste, containing at least 1000 ppm F, since this amount is effective in reducing dental caries in children [36].

Within the cycle of health care for pregnant women, prenatal consultation comprises major functions, such as health promotion, disease screening and diagnosis, as well as disease prevention. Thus, prenatal dental care promotes maternal and child health [37, 38]. However, dental prenatal care is still highly neglected by pregnant women due to the lack of knowledge of the real importance of this attention [39].

In addition, it is valid to understand the profile of pregnant women seeking dental care in order to promote adequate guidance and treatment [40]. A question to be addressed in consultations concerns the knowledge of pregnant women about their own oral health and the interference that this fact may have in the oral health of the child in the first years of life, and in the relationship with caries in early childhood, in addition to its future implications, such as impairing the cognitive development and quality of life of the child [41]. It is important to highlight that professionals act with an important role in the deconstruction of incorrect perceptions about dental care during pregnancy, and a pleasant, calm, and quiet conversation during consultations can amplify the commitment of pregnant women to oral health [42].

Environmental factors present in the gestational period (unbalanced diet, stress, exposure to smoking and alcohol) may have negative impacts on pregnant women's health indicators, such as excessive weight gain, hypertension, gestational diabetes, and periodontal disease, among other chronic diseases [43–45]. That can result in negative events, both at the end of pregnancy, as prematurity (<37 weeks), large babies for gestational age or fetal macrosomia (≥4000 g), or after birth, such as asthma, delayed neuropsychomotor development and other chronic diseases [46, 47].

Knowing this, the dentist, together with other health care providers, can guide pregnant women to a healthier lifestyle, since their attitudes and behaviors in these first 1000 days of life are determinants for a healthier pregnancy, with repercussions on the health of the pregnant woman and the health of the baby [48].

6. Oral health education and dental consultation

The deficiency of knowledge in oral health can favor the occurrence of diseases and lead to the worsening of existing problems [49]. The lack of information causes dental services to be used mainly in precarious or urgent dental conditions when it has some associated painful symptomatology [50].

There is a substantial incompatibility between the oral health needs of communities and the availability, location, and type of dental services provided [51]. In high- and middle-income countries, young children, low-income families, marginalized groups, and people living with disabilities are generally poorly served, especially when compared to the access of wealthy families to dental services [52–55]. The current model of dental care and preventive clinical policy does not meet the global burden of oral diseases [29]. Although there are concepts to integrate primary oral health care into primary health care, they have not beeh fully expanded, which contributes even more to the challenge of providing access to even primary oral health care [56]. With this, oral health and the dental profession have become somewhat isolated and marginalized from the main developments in health policies and health care systems [29].

In addition, several studies have shown that oral hygiene instruction, dietary guidance, brushing with fluoridated toothpaste, flossing, and periodic follow-up with the dentist, for preventive prophylaxis and treatment, significantly increased the number of caries-free children [57, 58]. Continuous and periodic preventive consultations are extremely important because only with follow-up is it possible to evaluate family dental risk factors; parents' education about tooth eruption; oral hygiene, breastfeeding, and dietary counseling; if necessary, to carry out interceptive and preventive treatment; and establish a positive relationship between the family and the dental team [59, 60].

Current scientific evidence shows that the success of caries prevention and treatment also lies in the assessment of the risk of caries in the patient, in changing the dental biofilm complex, and in modifying oral factors [61]. A validated tool that was created to represent the multifactorial nature of dental caries disease is the management of caries by risk assessment (CAMBRA), as it emphasizes the balance between pathological and protective factors in the caries process [62–65].

Thus, it is possible to identify pathological factors such as inadequate oral self-care practices, frequency of fluoride exposure in the intake of carbohydrates, cariogenic bacteria and history of caries, and also protective factors such as ideal exposure to fluoride, dietary control of sucrose and good oral hygiene habits [66]. Using the knowledge acquired with an assessment and risk of caries, the dentist can implement a change of behavior to reduce risk factors, and increase individualized and standardized protection factors for each patient, resulting in disease control [61].

It is important that the health professional is aware of these measures to demystify beliefs and reinforce the guidelines for the family about the oral health of babies, since they can have repercussions on the development and growth of the child [41]. The efficient mechanical removal of dental biofilm is essential for the prevention of caries in early childhood, for this, it is necessary to perform the hygiene of the child's mouth, after the first tooth eruption with a brush and fluoridated toothpaste [41]. Thus, the professional should make parents and caregivers aware that caries disease is a disease that can be prevented and that the adoption of healthy habits, such as a balanced diet, hygiene, and maintenance of oral health is fundamental to avoid its occurrence [17].

7. Conclusions

Based on the present study, it is concluded the importance of establishing the relationship between the dentist and the pregnant woman, since educational actions initiated early act directly on health in the gestational period and in the child's growth. The consumption of early sugar in children, that is, before 2 years of age is correlated with the occurrence of caries in early childhood, due to family habits. Therefore, it becomes relevant instructions that help in the maintenance of healthy nutritional habits, and correct oral hygiene practices, since focusing on these educational actions increases the chances of healthy pregnancy and child development.

Acknowledgements

The authors thank CAPES (doctoral scholarship to GCCL), University of Sao Paulo (PUB-USP undergraduate scholarship to LGF) and 5° Edital Santander/USP/FUSP de Fomento às Iniciativas de Cultura e Extensão da Pró-Reitoria de Cultura e Extensão Universitária (to FWGPS) for financial support.

Conflict of interest

The authors state that the literature review was conducted in the absence of commercial or financial relations that could be interpreted as a potential conflict of interest.

Author details

Luanna Gonçalves Ferreira, Giuliana de Campos Chaves Lamarque
and Francisco Wanderley Garcia Paula-Silva*
Department of Pediatric Clinics, School of Dentistry Ribeirão Preto, University of São Paulo, Ribeirão Preto, SP, Brazil

*Address all correspondence to: franciscogarcia@forp.usp.br

References

[1] Phantumvanit P, Makino Y, Ogawa H, et al. WHO global consultation on public health intervention against early childhood caries. Community Dentistry and Oral Epidemiology. 2018;**46**(3): 280-287. DOI: 10.1111/cdoe.12362

[2] Kilian M, Chapple IL, Hannig M, et al. The oral microbiome—An update for oral healthcare professionals. British Dental Journal. 2016;**221**(10):657-666. DOI: 10.1038/sj.bdj.2016.865

[3] Fejerskov O, Nyvad B, Kidd EA. Pathology of Dental Caries. Dental caries: The Disease and Its Clinical Management. 3rd ed. Oxford (UK): Wiley Blackwell; 2015. pp. 7-9

[4] Ribeiro CCC, Silva MCBD, Nunes AMM, et al. Overweight, obese, underweight, and frequency of sugar consumption as risk indicators for early childhood caries in Brazilian preschool children. International Journal of Paediatric Dentistry. 2017;**27**(6):532-539. DOI: 10.1111/ipd.12292

[5] World Health Organization. Guideline: Sugars Intake for Adults and Children. 2015. Available from: https://www.who.int/publications/i/item/9789241549028 [Accessed: April 15, 2021]

[6] World Health Organization. WHO Expert Consultation on Public Health Intervention against Early Childhood Caries: Report of a Meeting; January 26-28, 2016; Bangkok, Tailândia. 2017. Available from: https://apps.who.int/iris/handle/10665/255627 [Accessed: April 15, 2021]

[7] Seow WK, Leishman SJ, Palmer JE, et al. A longitudinal observational study of developmental defects of enamel from birth to 6 years of age. JDR Clinical Transaction Research. 2016;**1**(3):285-291. DOI: 10.1177/2380084416655744

[8] Pitts NB, Zero DT, Marsh PD, et al. Dental caries. Nature Reviews. Disease Primers. 2017;**3**:17030. DOI: 10.1038/nrdp.2017.30

[9] Machiulskiene V, Campus G, Carvalho JC, et al. Terminology of dental caries and dental caries management: Consensus Report of a Workshop Organized by ORCA and Cardiology Research Group of IADR. Caries Research. 2020;**54**(1):7-14. DOI: 10.1159/000503309

[10] Manton DJ. Child dental caries—A global problem of inequality. Eclinical Medicine. 2018;**1**:3-4

[11] American Academy of Pediatric Dentistry. Caries-risk Assessment and Management for Infants, Children, and Adolescents. The Reference Manual of Pediatric Dentistry. Chicago, IL: American Academy of Pediatric Dentistry; 2020. pp. 243-247

[12] Tinanoff N, Baez RJ, Diaz Guillory C, et al. Early childhood caries epidemiology, aetiology, risk assessment, societal burden, management, education, and policy: Global perspective. International Journal of Paediatric Dentistry. 2019;**29**(3):238-248. DOI: 10.1111/ipd.12484

[13] Ha DH, Do LG, Spencer AJ, et al. Factors influencing early feeding of foods and drinks containing free sugars—A birth cohort study. International Journal of Environmental Research and Public Health. 2017;**14**(10):1270. DOI: 10.3390/ijerph14101270

[14] Wang Y, Guglielmo D, Welsh JA. Consumption of sugars, saturated fat, and sodium among US children from infancy through preschool age, NHANES 2009-2014. The American Journal of Clinical Nutrition. 2018;**108**(4):868-877. DOI: 10.1093/ajcn/nqy168

[15] Chaffee BW, Feldens CA, Rodrigues PH, Vítolo MR. Feeding practices in infancy associated with caries incidence in early childhood. Community Dentistry and Oral Epidemiology. 2015;**43**(4):338-348. DOI: 10.1111/cdoe.12158

[16] Folayan MO, Oginni AB, El Tantawi M, et al. Association between nutritional status and early childhood caries risk profile in a suburban Nigeria community. International Journal of Paediatric Dentistry. 2020;**30**(6):798-804. DOI: 10.1111/ipd.12645

[17] Ha DH, Do LG. Early life professional and layperson support reduce poor oral hygiene habits in toddlers: A Prospective Birth Cohort Study. Dental Journal (Basel). 2018;**6**(4):56

[18] Marsh PD. In sickness and in health-what does the oral microbiome mean to us? An ecological perspective. Advanced Dental Résumé. 2018;**29**(1):60-65

[19] Proctor GB. The physiology of salivary secretion. Periodontology. 2016;**70**:11-25

[20] Mathur VP, Dhillon JK. Dental caries: A disease that needs attention. Indian Journal of Pediatrics. 2018;**85**(3):202-206. DOI: 10.1007/s12098-017-2381-6

[21] Rosier BT, Marsh PD, Mira A. Resilience of the oral microbiota in health: Mechanisms that prevent dysbiosis. Journal of Dental Research. 2018;**97**(4):371-380. DOI: 10.1177/0022034517742139

[22] Marshall TA. Dietary implications for dental caries: A practical approach on dietary counseling. Dental Clinics of North America. 2019;**63**(4):595-605

[23] Schwendicke F, Frencken JE, Bjorndal L, et al. Managing carious lesions: Consensus recommendations on carious tissue removal. Advances in Dental Research. 2016;**28**(2):58-67. DOI: 10.1177/0022034516639271

[24] Feldens CA, dos Santos IF, Kramer PF, Vítolo MR, et al. Early-life patterns of sugar consumption and dental caries in the permanent teeth: A Birth Cohort Study. Caries Research. 2021;**55**:505-514. DOI: 10.1159/000518890

[25] Peres MA, Sheiham A, Liu P, Demarco FF, Silva AE, Assunção MC, et al. Sugar consumption and changes in dental caries from childhood to adolescence. Journal of Dental Research. 2016;**95**(4):388-394. DOI: 10.1177/0022034515625907

[26] Heilmann A, Tsakos G, Watt RG. Oral health over the life course. In: Burton-Jeangros C, Cullati S, Sacker A, Blane D, editors. A Life Course Perspective on Health Trajectories and Transitions: Life Course Research and Social Policies. Vol. 4. Cham: Springer; 2015. pp. 39-59. DOI: 10.1007/978-3-319-20484-0_3

[27] Albino J, Tiwari T. Preventing childhood caries: A review of recent behavioral research. Journal of Dental Research. 2016;**95**(1):35-42. DOI: 10.1177/0022034515609034

[28] Anil S, Anand PS. Early childhood caries: Prevalence, risk factors, and prevention. Frontiers in Pediatrics. 2017;**5**:157. DOI: 10.3389/fped.2017.00157

[29] Peres MA, Macpherson LMD, Weyant RJ, et al. Oral diseases: A global public health challenge. Lancet. 2019;**394**(10194):249-260. DOI: 10.1016/S0140-6736(19)31146-8

[30] Dimaisip-Nabuab J, Duijster D, Benzian H, et al. Nutritional status, dental caries and tooth eruption in children: A longitudinal study in Cambodia, Indonesia and Lao PDR. BMC Pediatrics. 2018;**18**(1):300. DOI: 10.1186/s12887-018-1277-6

[31] Jordan AR, Becker N, Jöhren HP, Zimmer S. Early childhood caries and caries experience in permanent dentition: A 15-year Cohort Study. Swiss Dental Journal. 2016;**126**(2):114-119

[32] Nyvad B, Fejerskov O. The caries control concept. In: Fejerskov O, Nyvad B, Kidd E, editors. Dental Caries: The Disease and Its Clinical Management. Oxford: Wiley Blackwell; 2015. pp. 235-243

[33] Douglass AB, Douglass JM, Krol DM. Educating pediatricians and family physicians in children's oral health. Academic Pediatrics. 2009;**9**(6):452-456. DOI: 10.1016/j.acap.2009.09.004

[34] de Silva AM, Hegde S, Akudo Nwagbara B, et al. Community-based population-level interventions for promoting child oral health. Cochrane Database System. 2016;**9**(9):CD009837

[35] Levine R, Stillman-Lowe C. The Scientific Basis of Oral Health Education. Suíça: Springer International Publishing; 2019

[36] IAPD. Foundational Articles and Consensus Recommendations: Use of Fluoride for Caries Preventino. 2020. Available from: https://iapdworld.org/03_Use-of-Fluoride-for-Caries-Prevention.pdf [Accessed: December 15, 2021]

[37] Concha Sánchez S, Almario Barrera A, Pabón OH. Percepciones y factores asociados a la salud bucal y la atención odontológica en el periodo perinatal en las mujeres y sus bebés. Odontología Sanmarquina. 2020;**23**(3):241-251

[38] Saliba TA, Custódio LB, Saliba NA, et al. Dental prenatal care in pregnancy. RGO—Revista Gaúcha de Odontologia (Online). 2019;**67**:1-9

[39] Massoni ACLT, Pereira RB, Nóbrega DRM, et al. Avaliação do conhecimento de gestantes e puérperas primíparas e multíparas sobre cárie dentária. Revista Gaúcha de Odontologia. 2015;**63**(2):45-52

[40] Guidolini Martinelli K, Belotti L, Martins PY, et al. Fatores associados ao cuidado de saúde bucal durante a gravidez. Arquivos Em Odontologia (Online). 2020;**56**:1-9

[41] Duarte KM. M. Educação em Saúde Bucal no pré-natal e puerpério. Saúde Bucal na APS: urgências, doenças transmissíveis, gestantes e pessoas com deficiência. Cuidado em saúde bucal para gestantes e puérperas. São Luís: UFMA; UNA-SUS; 2020. pp. 1-16

[42] Nunes Neto RA, Frutuoso MFP. ORAL health and the care of pregnant women: Workshops as a strategy to problematize practices in basic health care in residents living in the peripheral areas of the hills in the city of Santos. Revista Gaúcha de Odontologia. 2018;**66**(4):305-316

[43] May PA, Hasken JM, Blankenship J, et al. Breastfeeding and maternal alcohol use: Prevalence and effects on child outcomes and fetal alcohol spectrum disorders. Reproductive Toxicology. 2016;**63**:13-21. DOI: 10.1016/j.reprotox.2016.05.002

[44] Abraham M, Alramadhan S, Iniguez C, et al. A systematic review of maternal smoking during pregnancy and fetal measurements with meta-analysis. PLoS One. 2017;**12**(2):e0170946. DOI: 10.1371/journal.pone.0170946

[45] Pietrobelli A, Agosti M, MeNu Group. Nutrition in the first 1000 days: Ten practices to minimize obesity emerging from published Science. International Journal of Environmental Research and Public Health. 2017;**14**(12):1491

[46] Gustavson K, Ystrom E, Stoltenberg C, et al. Smoking in pregnancy and child ADHD. Pediatrics. 2017;**139**(2):e20162509

[47] Nascimento JXPT, Ribeiro CCC, Batista RFL, et al. The First Days of Life Factors Associated with "Childhood Asthma Symptoms". London: Brisa Cohort; 2017

[48] Pereira SMDS, Ribeiro CCC. Os primeiros 1000 dias de vida como uma oportunidade para a prevenção das DCNT bucais e sistêmicas: o que o cirurgião-dentista precisa saber? Universidade Federal do Maranhão. Curso Saúde Bucal na Atenção Primária: urgências, doenças transmissíveis, gestantes e pessoas com deficiência. Assistência odontológica para pacientes com DCNT na Atenção Primária: doenças cardiovasculares. Assistência à saúde bucal para gestantes e puérperas. São Luís: UFMA; Curso Saúde Bucal na Atenção Primária: urgências, doenças transmissíveis, gestantes e pessoas com deficiência; 2020. pp. 1-19

[49] World Health Organization Health Promotion Glossary. 1998. Available from: https://www.who.int/healthpromotion/about/HPR%20Glossary%201998.pdf [Accessed: April 15, 2021]

[50] Gilbert GH, Duncan RP, Shelton BJ. Social determinants of tooth loss. Health Services Research. 2003;**38**(6 Pt 2):1843-1862. DOI: 10.1111/j.1475-6773.2003.00205.x

[51] Watt et al. Ending the neglect of global oral health: Time for radical action. Lancet. 2019;**394**(10194):261-272

[52] Blánaid D, Tim N, Paul B, Kate J. Oral health care needs and oral health-related quality of life (OHIP-14) in homeless people. Community Dental Oral Epidemiology. 2010;**38**(2):136-144

[53] Freitas DJ, Kaplan LM, Tieu L, Ponath C, Guzman D, Kushel M. Oral health and access to dental care among older homeless adults: Results from the HOPE HOME study. Journal of Public Health Dentistry. 2019;**79**(1):3-9. DOI: 10.1111/jphd.12288

[54] Kisely S, Quek LH, Pais J, Lalloo R, Johnson NW, Lawrence D. Advanced dental disease in people with severe mental illness: Systematic review and meta-analysis. The British Journal of Psychiatry. 2011;**199**(3):187-193. DOI: 10.1192/bjp.bp.110.081695

[55] Walsh T, Tickle M, Milsom K, Buchanan K, Zoitopoulos L. An investigation of the nature of research into dental health in prisons: A systematic review. British Dental Journal. 2008;**204**(12):683-689

[56] Cheer T, Hak S, Courtel F, Durward C. Improving the provision of the Basic Package of Oral Care (BPOC) in Cambodia. International Dental Journal. 2009;**59**(1):47-52

[57] Daou MH, Eden E, El Osta N. Age and reasons of the first dental visit of children in Lebanon. Journal of Medical Libanais. 2016;**64**(1):18-22

[58] Gomez SS, Weber AA, Emilson CG. A prospective study of a caries prevention program in pregnant women an their children five and six years of age. Journal of Dentistry for Children. 2001;**68**(3):191-195

[59] Gripp VC, Schlagenhauf U. Prevention of early mutans streptococci transmission in infants by professional tooth cleaning and chlorhexidine varnish treatment of the mother. Caries Research. 2002;**36**(5):366-372. DOI: 10.1159/000065958

[60] Bhaskar V, McGraw KA, Divaris K. The importance of preventive dental visits from a young age: Systematic review and current perspectives. Clinical, Cosmetic and Investigational Dentistry. 2014;**6**:21-27. DOI: 10.2147/CCIDE.S41499

[61] Kriegler K, Blue CM. Caries management by risk assessment vs. traditional preventive strategies: Effect on oral health behaviors and caries diagnoses: A Retrospective Case-Control Observational Design. Clinical Case Reports. 2021;**9**:e04751

[62] Featherstone JD. Caries prevention and reversal based on the caries balance. Pediatric Dentistry. 2006;**28**(2):128-132

[63] Featherstone JD. The science and practice of caries prevention. Journal of American Dental Association. 2000;**131**(7):887-899

[64] Takahashi N, Nyvad B. The role of bacteria in the caries process: Ecological perspectives. Journal of Dental Research. 2011;**90**(3):294-303. DOI: 10.1177/0022034510379602

[65] Featherstone JD, White JM, Hoover CI, Rapozo-Hilo M, et al. A randomized clinical trial of anticaries therapies targeted according to risk assessment (caries management by risk assessment). Caries Research. 2012;**46**(2):118-129. DOI: 10.1159/000337241

[66] Rechmann P, Chaffee BW, Rechmann BMT, Featherstone JDB. Changes in caries risk in a practice-based Randomized Controlled Trial. Advances in Dental Research. 2018;**29**(1):15-23. DOI: 10.1177/0022034517737022

Chapter 5

Caries Management Aided by Fluorescence-Based Devices

Atena Galuscan, Daniela Jumanca and Aurora Doris Fratila

Abstract

Fluorescence-based intraoral cameras are increasingly gaining more interest in the modern dental practice, as an aid for the early detection of carious lesions. Such devices can have different operating systems, such as infrared lasers, quantitative light fluorescence (QLF), or LED lights, but they all rely on the fluorescent properties of tooth structures. Healthy enamel and enamel affected by demineralization have different light-scattering properties, a fact that allows for distinction under excitation with light of a known wavelength. The central problem in the treatment of dental decay is that operational care is still considered the predominant management plan for caries control in the general practice. Devices that use fluorescence have the potential to improve the detection and management of carious lesions significantly. Currently, there are several intraoral devices that employ fluorescence on the market, but more validation studies would be required to uphold the interest of the newly developed devices and to justify their reliability in clinical practice. Dental professionals cannot yet solely rely on one single-fluorescence device for incipient caries diagnosis, but they already present themselves as useful adjunctive tools to traditional examination methods.

Keywords: caries, fluorescence, intraoral scanners, oral health, diagnosis, prevention, noninvasive

1. Introduction

The clinical diagnosis of caries, which uses visual inspection and radiographs, is an imperfect process, making the development of dental plaque more likely to occur [1]. Previous studies have shown that the traditional examination for caries has limited performance, especially in detecting dental caries in the early stages. Appropriate treatment of carious lesions demands detection at an early stage and minimally invasive cavity preparation in order to preserve the maximum natural tooth structure; nevertheless, dental caries is one of the most afflictions worldwide [2–4].

For the visual-tactile examination for caries detection, the International Caries Detection and Assessment System (ICDAS-II) is usually used. The system provides proper data collection and guarantees standardization; however, visual evaluation is always dependent on the evaluator. Therefore, providing an additional diagnostic tool in the dental practice allows for objective assessment of enamel demineralization beginning from its early stages.

In the last years, the interest in optical devices which use nonionizing radiation, allowing them to detect and monitor caries, has been growing. Among these, cutting-edge technologies are intraoral cameras that combine fluorescence detection systems [5].

2. Fluorescent properties of teeth

Fluorescence occurs when a material emits light of different wavelengths, after absorbing light of higher energy. Because of this difference in energy, the color of the emitted fluorescence light is always different than that of the excitation light (produced by a source of defined parameters), having a longer wavelength and lower photon energy, as a result of the absorption of energy by the examined material [6, 7]. Hence, violet or blue excitation light will cause emissions that are green, orange, or red (depending on the examined material), all of which are longer wavelengths of visible light. Similarly, red excitation will cause emissions in the near-infrared region. This occurrence is known as the Stokes' shift.

One of the most common bacteria associated with carious lesions is lactobacilli, which strongly emit visible red fluorescence; even stronger than the mutans streptococci. It has been generally acknowledged that red-light emission caused by violet light excitation is well suited for the detection of caries-associated pathogens, such as streptococci and lactobacilli. Because of this feature, a range of devices for caries detection started using 405 nm violet light-emitting diodes, including intraoral cameras [8, 9].

Another notable feature is the suitability of porphyrin molecules (such as protoporphyrin IX and coproporphyrin) as markers for identifying carious lesions, considering the fact that porphyrin derivates do not occur within healthy tooth surfaces. These molecules are, too, fluorophores with maximum excitation at around 405 nm. As soon as the initial stage of a carious lesion forms, red fluorescence is emitted by porphyrins. According to the literature, porphyrins emitted light over 570 nm with double peaks, which are characteristic of these molecules [10].

The number of fluorophores present in the examined area is linearly proportional to the emission intensity, the fluorescent property is thus a very useful tool for quantification [11].

Additionally, the Maillard reaction products are currently the best-known dental caries products. They manifest themselves through browning discoloration, being a nonenzymatic reaction between reducing sugars (carbohydrate) and amino acids (protein). The Maillard reaction has been thoroughly studied in the field of food chemistry, where it has been found to be responsible for characteristic changes, such as the browning of bread during baking. The exact molecular structure of the brown pigment is still unknown. The Maillard reaction in human tissues is often associated with the complications of diabetes and old age, which include vascular stiffening, atherosclerosis, and renal insufficiency [12].

The organic components of sound tooth structure are responsible for the even green fluorescence when under illumination with violet–blue light, and certain fluorophores, for instance, tryptophan, account for the regular fluorescence of healthy dentin.

Also, worth mentioning is the fact that dentin hard tissue presents a relatively higher number of chromophores, resulting in a much brighter fluorescence compared to enamel. A high concentration of the fluorophores that emit green light can further be found at the dentinoenamel junction [13].

The process in which the development of dental caries affects fluorescence has been studied and characterized by researchers of the Karolinska Institute in Sweden as early as the 1980s. They found that the reduction in green fluorescence during caries development is caused by the reduction of mineral contents and simultaneously rising water content in the enamel. As a result, this leads to changes in light-scattering properties. Hence, when the green fluorescence fades, white spot lesions for instance, which are usually below the diagnostic threshold, become detectable [14, 15].

As mentioned above, fluorescence can serve as a very useful tool for quantification. Areas with a decrease in fluorescence over 5% are considered lesions [16]. This property helps quantify images with loss of fluorescence concerning the adjoining healthy tissue. For instance, fluorescence images of enamel areas that present white spot lesions can be digitalized and the ratio between those areas and the healthy surface on the same tooth can then be quantified efficiently [17].

3. Importance of adjunctive methods

A growing body of literature has studied and evaluated the importance of early caries diagnosis in the past years. According to the World Health Organization (WHO), untreated tooth decay impacts almost half of the worldwide population (44%) as of 2020, making it the most common condition included in the Global Burden of Disease Study. Carious lesions were shown to be five times more common than asthma and seven times more likely than hay fever in children [18].

Unfortunately, there is still considerable uncertainty and even drawback, exhibited by professionals regarding preventive strategies, which have yet to be utilized efficiently. There could be several reasons for this, but the central problem is that operational care is still considered the predominant management plan for caries control in the general practice. This is negatively impacting aspects, such as caries epidemiology, patients' quality of life, and long-term preservation of healthy tooth structure among others [19].

An increasing number of research highlight the need for innovative and reliable detection methods in the early (pre-cavitated) stages of caries, pointing out that visual examination has been found to be effective in more "pronounced" stages. Because of this, more sensitive and accurate devices and technologies are being developed, for practitioners to detect initial carious lesions as efficiently as possible [20].

It has been suggested by Makhija in 2014 that around 96% of carious lesions in early stages could be efficiently treated with noninvasive interventions. These findings seem to be well-founded, taking into consideration the trend of modern dentistry, which strives toward minimally invasive therapy, early diagnosis, and treatment of caries being a top priority goal [21]. One of the major drawbacks to reaching this goal is the fact that caries treatment often occurs in more advanced stages, being based mainly on symptoms and clinical signs – thus making it inadequate for a non-invasive treatment plan [22]. Uncertainties in detecting early lesions can arise even in the ranks of experienced practitioners, an assumption that is very plausible and natural [23, 24]. Accordingly, using digital methods like fluorescence-based devices, can improve the early caries detection [25, 26].

4. Fluorescence-based devices

Fundamental considerations when using fluorescence-based systems are the differences between the fluorescent properties of healthy and carious tooth structure, the used light wavelengths, as well as the approach used in examining the emitted fluorescence.

4.1 Infrared lasers

The DIAGNOdent Pen (KaVo, Biberach, Germany) is made up of a handpiece, which uses a red laser diode emitting light of 655 nm wavelength. Both the red light of the diode and the consequent fluorescence are transported through optical fibers (**Figure 1**). The emitted fluorescence is filtered and quantified to display the mineralization level of the examined surface/structure ranging on a scale from 0 to 99, which is then displayed by the device on a screen, showing a numerical value only (**Table 1**).

According to research conducted on the diagnostic validity of the DIAGNOdent Pen, it showed a higher sensitivity than visual or radiographic examination methods, but at the same time, lower sensitivity values of detecting dentin compared with enamel lesions. Some care is required in the use of the DIAGNOdent Pen camera when conducting clinical studies, due to difficulties with stain- and plaque- confounding assessments, and perhaps further work is needed before it can be routinely used in clinical studies [27].

A more recent study in which 628 occlusal fissures were analyzed, revealed a wide intra- and inter-investigator variability (reproducibility) for the DIAGNOdent Pen, findings which remain controversial [28].

According to multiple studies, what we know now, is that the DIAGNOdent Pen is insufficiently correlated with caries depth and ineffective for monitoring lesions over time. Because there is still some ambiguity regarding the performance and accuracy of the DIAGNOdent Pen, dental professionals should not rely on this device alone, overall having a poor clinical relevance in modern practice [29–33].

It is confirmed by systematic reviews of the DIAGNOdent Pen that further scientific research and insight into the clinical use of the device are necessary [34–36].

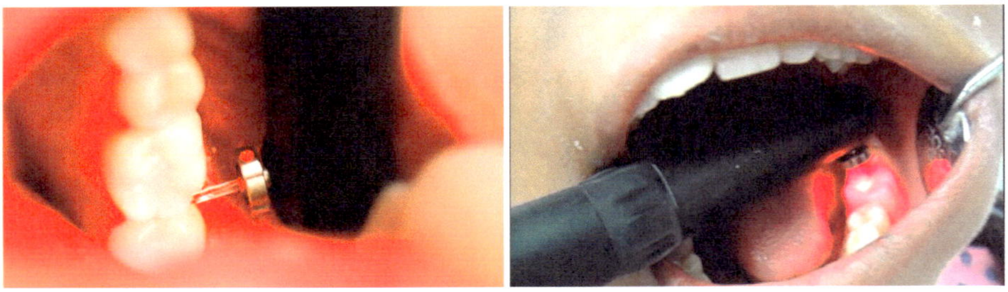

Figure 1.
DIAGNOdent pen in clinical use.

	Score	Meaning
Occlusal surfaces and pits	0–12	Healthy tissue
	13–24	Demineralized enamel
	>25	Dentine involved
Approximal surfaces	0–7	Healthy tissue
	8–15	Demineralized enamel
	>16	Dentine involved

Table 1.
Score scale of the DIAGNOdent pen according to the manufacturer.

4.2 Quantitative light fluorescence (QLF)

QLF consists of an intraoral camera with CCD (charge-coupled device) technology, which is a highly sensitive photon detector, connected to a light source emitting blue–green light. This technology targets the quantification of the mineral content of enamel, depending on changes in the fluorescence of sound versus carious enamel, after excitation at 405 nm. The fluorescence of the teeth is displayed on a screen, healthy enamel appearing green. The bacterial activity of porphyrin reaction where caries forms, results in surface changes, and thus, in light scattering, where carious lesions become visible. It is considered that a surface with demineralization over 5% can be called affected [37, 38]. QLF can measure fluorescence radiance loss in percent, as well as lesion size (mm2) to describe lesion severity, making it, according to a significant number of authors, suitable for prospective monitoring of tissue de- and remineralization.

Therefore, QLF has a great potential in being a supportive tool for monitoring the effects of preventive care on dental patients. Moreover, combining QLF with visual examination can significantly increase the sensitivity of detecting initial lesions [39, 40].

Several devices using QLF technology have been developed [41], which are as follows:

- Inspektor Pro (Inspektor Research Systems BV, Amsterdam, the Netherlands) (1st generation)
- Digital Biluminator 2+ device (QLF-D, Inspektor Research Systems BV) (2nd generation)
- Qraycam (AIOBIO, Seoul, Republic of Korea) (3rd generation)

4.3 LED cameras

A more recently developed caries detection system aided by fluorescence is the LED technology of certain intraoral cameras. This system illuminates the examined area of the tooth, records the emitted fluorescence, and intensifies the resulted image with the help of dedicated software. These devices include among others the intraoral camera VistaCam iX (Dürr Dental, Bietigheim-Bissingen, Germany), which operates using the software DBSWIN. The "Proof" interchangeable head displays carious lesions and plaque using fluorescence.

Similar to QLF systems, healthy enamel can be identified by its green fluorescence. The teeth are illuminated with violet light of 405 nm wavelength and the reflected fluorescent light is then filtered for light below 495 nm. The filtered light consists of the green color of healthy enamel with a peak at 510 nm, as well as the characteristic red fluorescence of cariogenic oral bacteria with a peak at 680 nm [42] (**Tables 2** and **3**).

A study carried out by Jablonski-Momeni et al. in which an experienced and a novice professional examined occlusal caries using the VistaProof, found that the fluorescence-based device showed high reproducibility and good diagnostic performance. Both examiners were able to use this system efficiently as a supportive means for caried monitoring, as well as diagnosis. Moreover, it also provided insightful visual and quantitative feedback to patients [43].

Rodrigues et al. presented similar results regarding the performance of the VistaCam iX, as well as the VistaProof [44].

Fluorescence color	Status	Score displayed
Green	Healthy enamel	0–1
Blue	Initial demineralization	1–1.5
Red	Deep enamel lesion/caries	1.5–2
Orange	Dentine lesion	2–2.5
Yellow	Deep dentine lesion	>2.5

Table 2.
Color code of the VistaCam iX according to the manufacturer.

VistaCam iX Display Status	VistaCam iX Fluorescence-Based Camera	Visual Caries Detection
0-1: Sound tissue; 1-1.5: Initial demineralization; 1.5-2.0: Deep enamel caries;	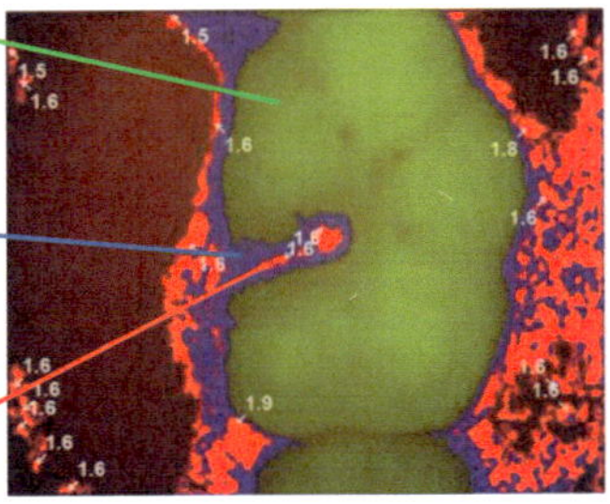	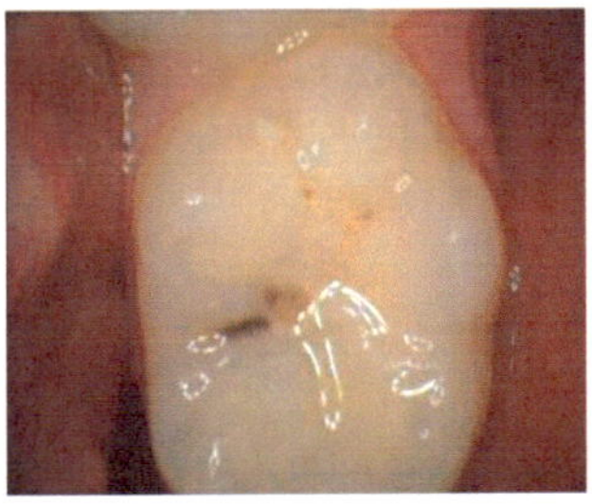
0-1: Sound tissue; 1-1.5: Initial demineralization; 1.5-2.0: Deep enamel caries;	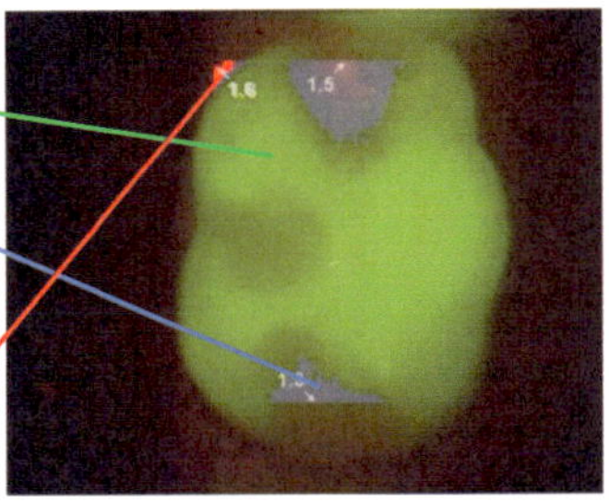	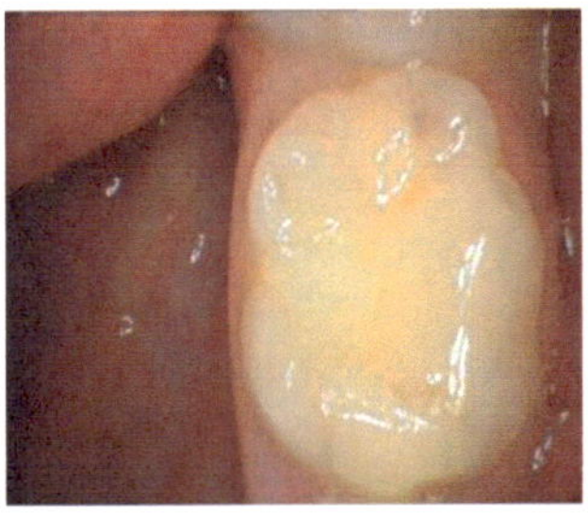

Table 3.
Description of visual and fluorescence-based diagnostic criteria with the VistaCam iX.

But one very recent study by Achilleos et al. (2021) has found that the use of neither the VistaProof device nor the DIAGNOdent Pen contributed to the incipient occlusal caries detection when compared to visual diagnosis criteria [13].

Another fluorescence-based device with an LED system is the SoproLife (Sopro-Acteon group, La Ciotat, France) intraoral camera. The practitioner can choose between two fluorescence modes of operating the camera:

- a diagnostic mode, in which the fluorescent colors are limited to those observed on the tooth
- a processing mode, in which the red of carious tissues is amplified, in order to guide the practitioner in eliminating the lesion

Additionally, there is a day-light mode, for intraoral photographs and videos.

The emitted blue light in fluorescence-mode is of 450 nm wavelength, thus healthy enamel appears green and carious lesions appear light to very dark red, similar to the VistaCam iX.

The image software enhances the emitted fluorescence of the examined surface (the tooth), allowing the practitioner to improve their visual inspection and decision-making [45].

The SoproLife camera allows observation of any variations in the optical properties to refine the caries diagnosis. It also provides more than a 50× magnification of the occlusal groove anatomy, to grant additional data on the carious potential of the examined tooth surface [46]. Although several authors consider the SoproLife camera a helpful tool in detecting and monitoring caries [47–50], others found no additional benefits in using this intraoral camera for detecting carious lesions in clinical practice [51].

More research is required, in order to facilitate the further development of these new systems and technologies, which should lead to improvements and better applicability in the modern and minimally invasive focused practice. Since there is currently a limited number of clinical research regarding the performance of fluorescence-based devices for caries diagnosis, especially for incipient carious lesions, values should be interpreted prudently until more clinically validated data is gathered through scientific studies.

5. Discussions

As modern dentistry is slowly shifting its focus on minimally invasive treatments and prevention is gaining more and more important in the day-to-day practice, there is no doubt that the constant development and innovation of new technologies is an essential step in this advance. This is also the reason we have chosen to review this particular topic, in order for recent graduates, young professionals, teachers, and even experienced practitioners to be up to date with research conducted on the accuracy and reliability of the currently available systems. Another reason would be to further raise awareness of the benefits and potential of new technologies for improving and easing the treatment quality. As observed in the present chapter, for all mentioned fluorescence-based devices, there are currently divided opinions and conclusions regarding their clinical relevance and benefit.

It is worth mentioning, that during the information gathering process for this chapter, a certain shortage of clinically relevant research conducted in the field of intraoral fluorescence cameras, in general, (but more striking, in the past years) has been noticed. It has occurred to us, that more validation studies are required to uphold the interest of the newly developed devices. Future studies should target the areas which require improvement for each device separately, after an extended period of clinical use, in order for companies to be able to improve said devices where necessary.

Fluorescence-based systems have a big potential in becoming an essential adjunctive tool for minimally intervention dentistry, enabling better detection of initial lesions and thereupon their remineralization. Nevertheless, it is of utter importance, for these, investigations to be continued and further parameters evaluated, for enhancement in their sensitivity, specificity, and reproducibility to aid the trustworthy and objective diagnosis of carious lesions.

6. Conclusions

We are confident that the fluorescence-based systems and devices used in dentistry will be further developed and improved, and they eventually will become meaningful tools in helping minimize the percentage of the population affected by dental caries significantly. Reducing operative care and increasing preventive care will have long-term benefits at levels for entire populations. Such devices even have the potential of becoming at-home monitoring tools for the dental plaque for patients, which then could lead to improved oral health.

The trend of minimally invasive and preventive dentistry has become remarkable in the past few years and this technology is truly revolutionary for modern oral health care.

Currently, we cannot solely rely only on one of the mentioned fluorescence devices, but they already present themselves as useful adjunctive tools for visual examination and radiography.

Conflict of interest

The authors declare no conflict of interest.

Author details

Atena Galuscan[1,2], Daniela Jumanca[1,2] and Aurora Doris Fratila[3*]

1 "Victor Babeş" University of Medicine and Pharmacy, Faculty of Dental Medicine, Timisoara, Romania

2 Translational and Experimental Clinical Research Center in Oral Health (TEXC-OH), Timisoara, Romania

3 Ludwig-Maximilian-University Munich, Faculty of Dental Medicine, München, Germany

*Address all correspondence to: a.fratila@campus.lmu.de

References

[1] Walsh LJ. Caries diagnosis aided by fluorescence. In: Arkanslan Z, editor. Dental Caries—Diagnosis and Management. Rijeka, Croatia: InTech Publishers; 2018. pp. 97-115

[2] Gimenez T, Piovesan C, Braga MM, Raggio DP, Deery C, Ricketts DN, et al. Visual inspection for caries detection: A systematic review and meta-analysis. Journal of Dental Research. 2015;**94**(7):895-904

[3] Braga MM, Mendes FM, Ekstrand KR. Detection activity assessment and diagnosis of dental caries lesions. Dental Clinics. 2010;**54**(3):479-493

[4] Hoskin ER, Keenan AV. Can we trust visual methods alone for detecting caries in teeth? Evidence-Based Dentistry. 2016;**17**(2):41-42

[5] Shakibaie F, Walsh LJ. Effect of oral fluids on dental caries detection by the VistaCam. Clinical and Experimental Dental Research. 2015;**1**(2):74-79

[6] Lee YK. Fluorescence properties of human teeth and dental calculus for clinical applications. Journal of Biomedical Optics. 2015;**20**(4):040901

[7] Hermanson AS, Bush MA, Miller RG, Bush PJ. Ultraviolet illumination as an adjunctive aid in dental inspection. Journal of forensic sciences. 2008;**53**(2):408-411

[8] Buchalla W, Lennon ÁM, Attin T. Comparative fluorescence spectroscopy of root caries lesions. European Journal of Oral Sciences. 2004;**112**(6):490-496

[9] Buchalla W, Lennon AM, Attin T. Fluorescence spectroscopy of dental calculus. Journal of Periodontal Research. 2004;**39**(5):327-332

[10] Slimani A, Nouioua F, Panayotov I, Giraudeau N, Chiaki K, Shinji Y, et al. Porphyrin and pentosidine involvement in the red fluorescence of enamel and dentin caries. International Journal of Experimental Dental Science 2016;**5**(1):1-0

[11] Timoshchuk MA, Ridge JS, Rugg AL, Nelson LY, Kim AS, Seibel EJ. Real-time porphyrin detection in plaque and caries: A case study. InLasers in Dentistry XXI. SPIE. Feb 24 2015;**9306**:48-58

[12] Kleter GA. Discoloration of dental carious lesions (a review). Archives of Oral Biology. 1998;**43**(8):629-632

[13] Achilleos E, Rahiotis C, Kavvadia K, Vougiouklakis G. In vivo validation of Diagnodent and vista proof devices vs ICDAS clinical criteria on incipient carious lesions in adults. Photodiagnosis and Photodynamic Therapy. 2021;**34**:102252

[14] Bjelkhagen H. Early detection of enamel caries by the luminescence excited by visible laser light. Swedish Dental Journal. 1982;**6**(1):1-7

[15] Sundström F, Fredriksson K, Montan S, Hafström-Björkman U, Ström J. Laser-induced fluorescence from sound and carious tooth substance: Spectroscopic studies. Swedish Dental Journal. 1985;**9**(2):71-80

[16] Achilleos EE, Rahiotis C, Kakaboura A, Vougiouklakis G. Evaluation of a new fluorescence-based device in the detection of incipient occlusal caries lesions. Lasers in Medical Science. 2013;**28**(1):193-201

[17] Van der Veen MH, de Jong ED. Application of quantitative light-induced fluorescence for assessing early caries

lesions. Monographs in Oral Science. 2000;**17**:144-162

[18] Kopycka-Kedzierawski DT, Bell CH, Billings RJ. Prevalence of dental caries in early head start children as diagnosed using teledentistry. Pediatric Dentistry. 2008;**30**(4):329-333

[19] Gomez J. Detection and diagnosis of the early caries lesion. BMC Oral Health. 2015;**15**(1):1-7

[20] Zenhom Abd El Rahman SM, Ibrahim SH. Reliability of fluorescent camera versus visual assessment IN diagnosis of OCCUSAL carious lesion IN adult patients: INVIVO diagnostic study. Egyptian Dental Journal. 2021;**67**(1) January (Conservative Dentistry and Endodontics:823-833

[21] Makhija SK, Gilbert GH, Funkhouser E, Bader JD, Gordan VV, Rindal DB, et al. Twenty-month follow-up of occlusal caries lesions deemed questionable at baseline: Findings from the National Dental Practice-Based Research Network. The Journal of the American Dental Association. 2014;**145**(11):1112-1118

[22] Nyvad B. Diagnosis versus detection of caries. Caries Research. 2004;**38**(3):192-198

[23] Holtzman JS, Ballantine J, Fontana M, Wang A, Calantog A, Benavides E, et al. Assessment of early occlusal caries pre-and post-sealant application—An imaging approach. Lasers in Surgery and Medicine. 2014;**46**(6):499-507

[24] Rodrigues JA, Lussi A, Seemann R, Neuhaus KW. Prevention of crown and root caries in adults. Periodontology 2000. 2011;**55**(1):231-249

[25] Meyer-Lueckel H. In: Paris S, Ekstrand KR, Effenberger S, editors. Caries Management: Science and Clinical Practice. Stuttgart: Thieme; 2013

[26] Thanh MT, Van Toan N, Toan DT, Thang NP, Dong NQ, Dung NT, et al. Diagnostic value of fluorescence methods, visual inspection and photographic visual examination in initial caries lesion: A systematic review and meta-analysis. Dentistry Journal. 2021;**9**(3):30

[27] Luczaj-Cepowicz E, Marczuk-Kolada G, Obidzinska M, Sidun J. Diagnostic validity of the use of ICDAS II and DIAGNOdent pen verified by micro-computed tomography for the detection of occlusal caries lesions—An in vitro evaluation. Lasers in Medical Science. 2019;**34**(8):1655-1663

[28] Terrer E, Slimani A, Giraudeau N, Levallois B, Tramini P, Bonte E, et al. Performance of fluorescence-based systems in early caries detection: A public health issue. The Journal of Contemporary Dental Practice. 2019;**20**:1126-1131

[29] Lussi A, Hack A, Hug I, Heckenberger H, Megert B, Stich H. Detection of approximal caries with a new laser fluorescence device. Caries Research. 2006;**40**(2):97-103

[30] Ghaname ES, Ritter AV, Heymann HO, Vann WF Jr, Shugars DA, Bader JD. Correlation between laser fluorescence readings and volume of tooth preparation in incipient occlusal caries in vitro. Journal of Esthetic and Restorative Dentistry. 2010;**22**(1):31-39

[31] Abrams SH, Sivagurunathan KS, Silvertown JD, Wong B, Hellen A, Mandelis A, et al. Correlation with caries lesion depth of the canary system, DIAGNOdent and ICDAS II. The Open Dentistry Journal. 2017;**11**:679

[32] Hamilton JC, Gregory WA, Valentine JB. DIAGNOdent measurements and correlation with the depth and volume of minimally invasive cavity preparations. Operative Dentistry. 2006;**31**(3):291-296

[33] Teo TK, Ashley PF, Louca C. An in vivo and in vitro investigation of the use of ICDAS, DIAGNOdent pen and CarieScan PRO for the detection and assessment of occlusal caries in primary molar teeth. Clinical oral investigations. 2014;**18**(3):737-744

[34] Slimani A, Terrer E, Manton DJ, Tassery H. Carious lesion detection technologies: Factual clinical approaches. British Dental Journal. 2020;**229**(7):432-442

[35] Bader JD, Shugars DA. A systematic review of the performance of a laser fluorescence device for detecting caries. The Journal of the American Dental Association. 2004;**135**(10):1413-1426

[36] Khandelwal A, Jose J, Ajitha P. Early Detection of Dental Caries–A Review. Available from: https://www.researchgate.net/profile/Akshay-Khandelwal-5/publication/347885878_Early_detection_of_dental_caries_-A_review/links/5fe58959a6fdccdcb8fc092c/Early-detection-of-dental-caries-A-review.pdf

[37] Kühnisch J, Heinrich-Weltzien R. Quantitative light-induced fluorescence (QLF)--a literature review. International Journal of Computerized Dentistry. 2004;7(4):325-338

[38] Zandoná AF, Santiago E, Eckert G, Fontana M, Ando M, Zero DT. Use of ICDAS combined with quantitative light-induced fluorescence as a caries detection method. Caries Research. 2010;**44**(3):317-322

[39] Fathima F, Mathew BT. Quantitative light-induced fluorescence (QLF) IN orthodontics–a review. European Journal of Molecular & Clinical Medicine. 2021;**8**(3):303-312

[40] Higham SM, Pretty IA, Edgar WM, Smith PW. The use of in situ models and QLF for the study of coronal caries. Journal of Dentistry. 2005;**33**(3):235-241

[41] Park SW, Kim SK, Lee HS, Lee ES, de Jong ED, Kim BI. Comparison of fluorescence parameters between three generations of QLF devices for detecting enamel caries in vitro and on smooth surfaces. Photodiagnosis and Photodynamic Therapy. 2019;**25**:142-147

[42] Eberhart J, Frentzen M, Thoms M. New optical techniques for caries detection-fluorescence based systems to identify Noncavitated lesions. ZWR. 2007;**116**(4):148-156

[43] Jablonski-Momeni A, Schipper HM, Rosen SM, Heinzel-Gutenbrunner M, Roggendorf MJ, Stoll R, et al. Performance of a fluorescence camera for detection of occlusal caries in vitro. Odontology. 2011;**99**(1):55-61

[44] Rodrigues JA, Hug I, Diniz MB, Lussi A. Performance of fluorescence methods, radiographic examination and ICDAS II on occlusal surfaces in vitro. Caries Research. 2008;**42**(4):297-304

[45] Guerrieri A, Gaucher C, Bonte E, Lasfargues JJ. Minimal intervention dentistry: Part 4. Detection and diagnosis of initial caries lesions. British Dental Journal. 2012;**213**(11):551-557

[46] Terrer E, Koubi S, Dionne A, Weisrock G, Sarraquigne C, Mazuir A, et al. A new concept in restorative dentistry: Light-induced fluorescence evaluator for diagnosis and treatment. Part 1: Diagnosis and

treatment of initial occlusal caries. The Journal of Contemporary Dental Practice. 2009;**10**(6):E086-E094

[47] Kockanat A, Unal MU. In vivo and in vitro comparison of ICDAS II, DIAGNOdent pen, CarieScan PRO and SoproLife camera for occlusal caries detection in primary molar teeth. European Journal of Paediatric Dentistry. 2017;**18**(2):99-104

[48] Zeitouny M, Cuisinier F, Tassery H, Fayyad-Kazan H. The efficacy of Soprolife® in detecting in vitro remineralization of early caries lesions. Journal of Oral & Maxillofacial Research. Apr 2020;**11**(2):11206

[49] Kotlow L. 7 SoproLife dental caries detection system. Microinvasive Dentistry: Clinical Strategies and Tools; 2020. p. 55

[50] Muller-Bolla M, Joseph C, Pisapia M, Tramini P, Velly AM, Tassery H. Performance of a recent light fluorescence device for detection of occlusal carious lesions in children and adolescents. European Archives of Paediatric Dentistry. 2017;**18**(3):187-195

[51] Theocharopoulou A, Lagerweij MD, van Strijp AJ. Use of the ICDAS system and two fluorescence-based intraoral devices for examination of occlusal surfaces. European Journal of Paediatric Dentistry. 2015;**16**(1):51-55

Chapter 6

Atraumatic Restorative Treatment: More than a Minimally Invasive Approach?

Manal A. Ablal

Abstract

Minimally invasive (MI) caries management has largely evolved over the years to include approaches that not only aimed to preserve as much tooth structure as possible but also to embrace prevention and risk management strategies. The atraumatic restorative treatment (ART) is a minimally invasive approach that was initially established to address the issue of increasing number of salvable teeth that kept being extracted in remote parts of the world where there was a limited access to the necessary equipment to enable preserving teeth in the primary and permanent dentitions. Managing carious lesions following ART is not as demanding as that in the conventional restorative methods, however, there are certain factors known to contribute to the failure of atraumatic restorative treatment that need to be considered to ensure success. However, and despite the advantages associated with using ART there seems to be a lack of awareness among dental practitioners regarding adopting this approach that can largely affect effective practice. Therefore, there is a need to spread the awareness and further educate practitioners particularly in this Covid-19 era where the virus and its variants have impacted the provision of routine dental treatment and will continue to do so for the foreseeable future.

Keywords: minimally invasive, atraumatic restorative treatment, caries management, sealants and restorations

1. Introduction

Dental caries is a widespread multifactorial oral disease where aetiological factors such as dietary carbohydrates, acidogenic microbial flora, time in addition to other specific host factors can greatly contribute to its development and progression [1, 2]. If left untreated, the complications of dental caries can affect oral as well as general health; both can eventually have a negative impact on human's quality of life [1]. The management of caries has traditionally involved drilling and the complete removal of all carious tissue which is then replaced by a restorative material [3]. This 'drill and fill' approach is not risk free though and often associated with either iatrogenic or caries-induced pulpal exposure, the incidence of which is greatly increased in deciduous and young adult teeth [3]. Other risks include the inevitable removal of sound tooth structure in the process of eliminating the carious lesion in addition to those risks related to the prolonged procedure times and the need for the local anaesthetic, that both can trigger dental anxiety [4]. Moreover, previous research into 'no drill' management techniques have stated that the 'drill & fill' approach is not required in many cases of dental caries as caries develops slowly and it could take the disease an average of 4–8 years to progress from enamel to dentine providing clinicians with sufficient time to detect and treat the lesion before it is cavitated and therefore, reducing the need for restorative treatment [5]. Therefore, there is a need for further emphasis on establishing more strategies such as minimal intervention approaches to effectively manage dental caries by intercepting the disease at its early stages while preventing the formation of new lesions [6, 7].

Minimal intervention (MI) is a branch of dentistry that aims at maintaining as much healthy tooth structure as possible through focusing on managing caries using a therapeutic or a biological approach rather than the traditional G.V Black operative guiding principles [8]. Minimally intervention dentistry (MID) is therefore based on four core principles (1) Early caries detection and assessment of potential risk factors. (2) Control of risk factors to either eliminate or minimise caries through the analysis of diet and lifestyle habits. (3) Arrest or remineralise early lesions using topical agents containing elements such as Fluorides and Calcium. (4) Remove caries conservatively, when intervention is required, to preserve as much sound tooth structure and maintain lifetime function [9].

MID has gained dental practitioners' interest worldwide, however, in areas such as developing countries where limited access to dental resources existed, there was a need to find alternative MI approaches to enable providing dental care to patients who are deemed suitable to receive minimally invasive treatments; hence, Atraumatic Restorative Treatment (ART) was developed [10, 11].

2. Atraumatic Restorative Treatment (ART)

ART is defined as the removal of demineralised soft dentine with the aid of hand instruments only followed by the replacement of the excavated tissues and sealing the adjacent pits and fissures using bonding or adhesive restorative materials [10, 11]. Although ART is an alternative approach to MID, it still encompasses the same MID core principles [9] and it can be used to conservatively manage caries in both primary and permanent dentitions particularly for patients who are considered suitable to have the procedure but are dentally anxious or challenging to handle [12, 13]. Other advantages to adopting ART include the removal of soft demineralised dentine; pits and fissures as well as the cavity get sealed with the restorative material; little or no pain is usually associated therefore, minimising the need for the local anaesthetic, greatly reduced patient stress as no vibrations from rotary instruments, infection control measures are simpler to follow, in addition to the relative low costs when compared to the conventional treatment modalities [11, 14].

3. Indications and contraindications of ART

As mentioned earlier, ART is indicated where there is a limited or no access to routine dental and preventive care, additionally it can be used as a community measure to control caries in schools or in care homes and for people with disability who are known to feel fear for dentists and dental treatments [15–18]. This approach is however contraindicated when there are signs of irreversible pulpitis, pulp exposure, presence of abscess, a sinus or a periapical/interradicular pathology or simply when lesions are inaccessible to hand instruments [18].

4. ART patient satisfaction and popularity among dental practitioners

According to previous studies, high satisfaction rates were received when 68% and 85% of the respective 5- to 18-year-old patients reported absence of pain during caries excavation and during filling [19]. Further research in patient perception of ART demonstrated that only 6 (6.6%) and 26 (29.2%) of the ninety 14- to 15-year-old students who accepted to be treated using the ART approach did experience pain and discomfort [20]. More supporting data were received, particularly from patients who previously received conventional restorative treatment that, of the 262 participated in the study, 99% expressed their satisfaction with ART restorations, 96.6% were willing to undergo this procedure in future, and 94.9% were happy to recommend this treatment approach to close relatives [21].

Existing research reported that the ART approach has already been used by most dental practitioners whenever they temporise teeth [22]. However, a later study that investigated the awareness of the ART method among 600 UK GDPs has concluded that only 42% indicated their awareness of the effectiveness of ART in the treatment of caries and that less than 10% of the participated GDPs used the 'true' ART technique [23].

5. Caries removal in ART

Dentine caries consists of two layers; the closer to the enamel outer infected (contaminated) and the deeper inner affected (non-contaminated) dentine [24]. The former layer is formed of dead, very soft tissue and therefore easy to excavate using hand instruments while the latter layer has a firmer consistency as it contains higher mineral content, sensitive as its formed by vital dentine, contains minimal or no bacteria and hence can be left behind to remineralise [25]. A common challenge encountered by dentists is how much contaminated dentine to be removed or retained in order to allow for pulp healing? The clinical differentiation between the two dentine layers is subjective, however, there has been a general consensus towards leaving some contaminated dentine in deep carious lesions as long as it is well-sealed within the cavity [26, 27]. This paradigm shift in understanding the carious process constitutes the basis of ART by changing the cariogenic environment through isolating caries bacteria from the biofilm of the oral cavity would result in enhancing the dentine-pulp complex defence mechanisms leading to slowing or arresting the deep carious lesions [28].

In an attempt to facilitate the decision of what strategy to adopt, ART Vs conventional, when removing carious tissue in asymptomatic teeth having noncleanable carious lesions with vital pulp and no signs of irreversible pulpitis, previous research reported that carious lesion depth (as demonstrated during radiographic assessment if justified) and the dentition type (primary vs permanent) can be taken as a guide in the decision-making process [29]. In the same study, the authors stated that the ART approach can be used to treat:

1. Primary and permanent teeth with shallow to moderate carious lesion depth that has not reached 1/3 or 1/4 of the dentine and having no risk of pulpal exposure.

2. Permanent teeth having deep carious lesions that has reached 1/3 or 1/4 of the dentine and showing risks of pulpal exposure.

Furthermore, in ART, once caries is excavated to firm in shallow to moderate cavities and to soft dentine in deep lesions, the excavated tissue is replaced as well as the adjacent pits and fissures are sealed using high viscosity glass ionomer cement or with a resin sealant [25] as will be described in the following sections.

6. Materials used in ART

Generally speaking, the minimally invasive concept is mainly about preserving as much tooth structure as possible indicating that the resultant cavity preparation in most situations does not conform to the ideal properties of including mechanical features for retention purpose. However, the advances in adhesive restorative materials enabled promoting MID and other approaches that fall under the MI umbrella namely ART.

The ART materials of choice are resin composites or glass ionomer cements (GICs), however, owing to its physical and chemical properties, GIC has mostly been indicated for use as ART sealant [12, 30]. Some of those properties are adhesion to enamel and dentine [31], anticariogenic effect due to fluoride release [32, 33], biocompatibility [34], coefficient of thermal expansion that is similar to enamel and dentine [35] in addition to the ease of manipulation and its relatively low cost. Several studies, however, have indicated that the viscosity of GIC is an equally important factor in the success of atraumatic restorative treatments with a wider agreement that high viscosity GIC (HVGIC) such as GC Fuji IX™ and 3M ESPE Ketac Molar™ are more durable than the low- or medium-viscosity namely GC Fuji lining™ LC and Ionofil Plus VOCO, respectively [36–40]. The reduced viscosity formulae were used in the early years following the introduction of ART technique; however, studies have reported that the material in both consistencies exhibited low wear resistance and lack of compressive strength in high stress-bearing areas [41, 42]. This has led manufacturers to develop an advanced GIC formula; the so-called HVGIC which characterised by having a high powder-to-liquid ratio and improved mechanical properties such as wear performance, compressive strength, and marginal adaptability rendering it more appropriate for use with ART [43–45]. Resin modified GIC (RMGIC) has also shown a promising performance than the conventional GIC as an ART sealant demonstrating highly acceptable retention rates in occlusal and approximal cavities which indicated that it can be considered as an alternative restorative material comparable to HVGIC in ART [46–48]. RMGIC is a two-component system: the conventional GIC acid-base in the form of Polyalkenoic acid and fluoro-aluminosilicate glass in addition to the resin and the light-initiating compound [49]. Similar to that of the conventional GIC, the resin-modified formula provides the cariostatic effect while possessing strength and better aesthetics from the resin content [49]. Furthermore, RMGIC has superior mechanical and physical properties to those of the conventional GIC enabling the material to provide increased fracture resistance in high occlusal load areas [50]. On the other hand, the presence of resin among the constituents indicates the potential risk of polymerisation shrinkage that could affect the material adaptation around the cavity walls and margins [51]. Other RMGIC disadvantages include marginal discolouration overtime [52], the increased cost when compared to the conventional GIC in addition to the inability to use RMGIC as an ART sealant when there are no light-cure equipment available [51].

Composite resin (CR) is another alternative material that can be used as an ART sealant restoration as previous research reported that CR used in ART approach showed good results similar to those from HVGIC [53]. The development in the adhesive material industry provided the new CR materials with much improved physical and mechanical properties such as flexural, tensile, and compressive strengths making them more suitable in areas inside the mouth which are under high occlusal stresses [54]. However, the inherent polymerisation shrinkage (PS) property and material handling are issues that can affect their longevity long term. Previous reports have shown that the volumetric shrinkage that results from the PS caused polymerisation stresses to pull restoration and the cavity walls towards the centre of the cavity which could eventually lead to poor internal and marginal adaptation resulting in microleakage and postoperative sensitivity [55, 56]. Furthermore, composite resin properties were enhanced to bond to caries-free dentine indicating that, when used as part of ART in deep cavities, the material will have lower bond strength to the soft dentine [29]. Therefore, when performing ART special care should be taken while excavating caries in moderate to deep lesions in the permanent dentition to leave behind soft dentine only on the pulpal floor whereas the cavity walls should be cleaned to ensure good marginal seal [29]. Additionally, it has also been recommended that placing CR in increments, rather than bulk fill, would help minimising the effect of PS [51]. Others, on the other hand, have found that using RMGIC as a liner in deep cavities under CR further reduced the effect of PS as RMGIC's lower modulus of elasticity enables it to absorb PS and occlusal loading stresses [50]. Despite all that, the multilayer placement and achieving high levels of moisture control when using composite resins make the use of HVGIC as an ART sealant restoration is the preferred option.

Compomers; resin reinforced glass ionomers have also been used as ART restorations as, similar to GIC, their cariostatic property due to the fluoride release provides an advantage to use them over composites particularly in primary teeth and high caries risk patients [57]. When their survival rates were tested against those of HVGIC, the two showed comparable results and both materials were suitable as occlusal and approximal restorations for ART in primary molars [58, 59]. However, due to their resin content compomers undergo some PS which could result in marginal leakage [60] and therefore, HVGIC remains the material of choice as an ART sealant restoration.

7. A step-by-step guide to ART sealants and restorations

The atraumatic restorative treatment approach is of two components: the ART sealants and ART restorations where in the former the pits and fissures get sealed using HVGIC while in the latter the excavated carious dentine is replaced with a sealant restoration [61]. It should be borne in mind though that with ART restorations, not only the cavity created as a result of carious dentine excavation gets filled with a sealant restoration, but the adjacent pits and fissure should be included in the sealing process [62, 63]. Pits and fissures of the posterior teeth are more prone to develop caries and sealing them provides a smooth protective layer that prevents food accumulation and bacterial growth in addition to facilitating maintaining those areas clean [64, 65].

Although it might sound simple and straightforward to perform, ART success is dependent on strictly following a set of steps and a prevention plan to ensure achieving the desired outcomes. The WHO Oral Health Programme has reported that ART is an important element of a health care package that includes promotion of oral health and prevention care [66]. Infection control measures should always be applied before, during and after the procedure. The next step would be to assess the carious lesion to ensure suitability for the ART approach; it has been reported that asymptomatic teeth with no signs of irreversible pulpits but having lesions extending into dentine where cavities are accessible to hand instruments are good candidates for ART [67]. Also, the ART approach can be used to restore one-and multi-surface cavities in the anterior as well as posterior teeth where the stages involved in cavity preparation and restoration are similar [67]. Achieving moisture control through the use of rubber dam, particularly while placing sealant restoration has always been recommended whenever applicable.

However, as the material mostly used for ART is GIC the use of rubber dam is not considered critical to the success of the procedure as studies have found no difference in the survival rates of ART restorations with or without its use [68] and therefore, the use of cotton wool rolls would be sufficient as long as they keep the surrounding area dry.

Since its initiation back in mid-80s, ART approach did not rely on using high technology equipment, but it rather simplified caries treatment to dental care providers in the developing countries to provide better oral health care to patients. One example is the no need for dental chairs as this approach was meant to enable dental practitioners to use ART in different field conditions such schools [69]. Nonetheless, good working conditions in terms of operator, assistant if available, and patient positions must be ensured for convenience and better treatment outcomes.

8. Armamentarium

One of the fundamental aspects of ART is the use of basic dental instruments and materials that can be found and easily handled in any non-high technology or even outside dental settings such as schools or nursing homes [63]. These include the following:

8.1 Basic dental instruments

- Mouth mirror
- Explorer/probe
- Spoon excavators (preferably different sizes)
- Dental Hatchet
- Tweezers
- Applier/carver
- Mixing pad and a spatula

8.2 Materials

- Glass Ionomer Cement (GIC)—High viscosity
- Dentine conditioning
- Cotton wool rolls and pellets
- Petroleum jelly/vaseline
- Mylar/plastic matrix strips for multi-surface restorations
- Wedges

9. Positioning and posture during ART procedure

Patient, dentist, and the assistant positions play an important role in facilitating the delivery of ART stages and could indirectly contribute to enhancing the success of the treatment. The below can be taken as a guide, however, depending on the patient's clinical presentation slight variations might be acceptable as long as the team is still adhering to practising safe dentistry.

9.1 Patient position

The patient should preferably be lying flat with suitable headrest to allow saliva to collect towards the back of the mouth to aid in achieving a dry field would work the best [16, 67]. The patient can then assist the operator in either turning the head sideways, tilting back- or forwards as required, and in having the mouth either fully or partially opened to facilitate delivery of procedure stages [67].

9.2 Operator position

Operators should continue complying with the standard dentist seating positions and posture [14, 16, 67]. With as much straight back as possible, the operator should be sitting behind the patient's head which can be slightly tilted depending on the quadrant and teeth surface.

9.3 Assistant position

When available, the assistant must sit to the left of a right-handed operator and sufficiently close to the patient to avoid leaning forward but at the same time should be approximately 10 cm higher than the operator to avoid having a restricted view. That position would also facilitate them reaching and transferring instruments and materials to the operator in the transfer zone [70].

10. The key stages involved in ART

As mentioned, ART can be used as either a preventative approach to seal caries susceptible pits and fissures or to restore early caries and simultaneously seal adjacent pits and fissures [16, 36, 37, 67]:

10.1 ART sealants using HVGIC to seal pits and fissures

1. The tooth undergoing treatment is to be isolated using cotton wool rolls and any food debris or plaque deposits removed from the pits and fissures using either a probe or a toothbrush (**Figure 1-1**).

2. Apply the dentine conditioner to the pits and fissures then wash off using a wet cotton pellet.

3. Cotton pellets are used to dry the occlusal surface.

4. HVGIC is mixed and applied to pits & fissures using the applier end of the instrument (**Figure 1-2**).

5. Pressure (press-finger technique) applied onto the occlusal surface using a lubricated finger for a few seconds until the GIC has initially set (**Figure 1-3**).

6. Remove finger and check that GIC has filled all pits and fissures then remove excess.

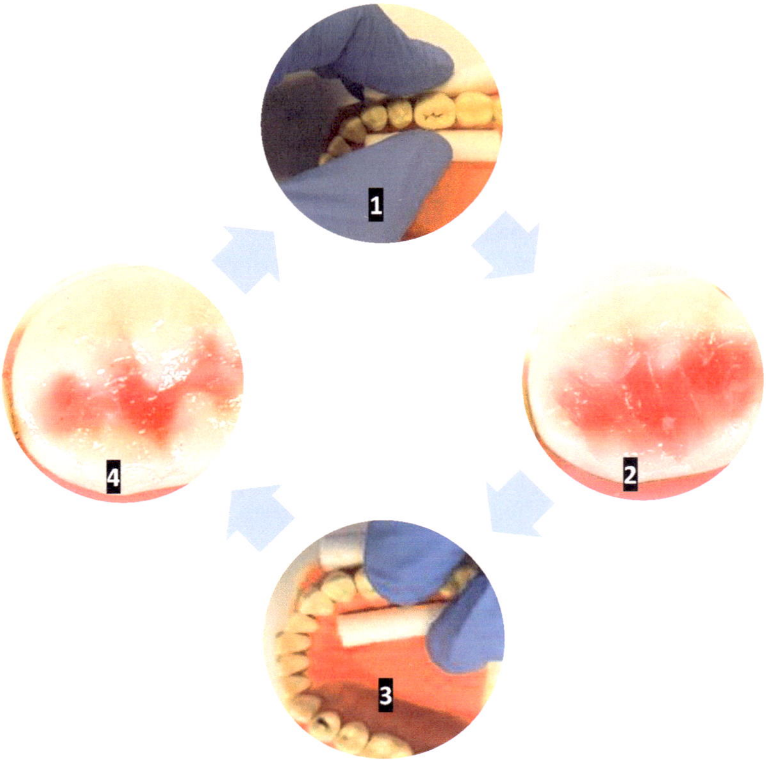

Figure 1.
Schematic representation of the steps involved in sealing non-cavitated fissures using HVGIC. In a clockwise direction: (1) Cotton wool roll isolated and debris free pits and fissure. (2) HVGIC placed over pits & fissures. (3) Finger- press over filled pits & fissures. (4) Adjusted and finished restoration.

7. Check occlusion and adjust if necessary.

8. Place a fresh layer of petroleum jelly on the occlusal surface (**Figure 1-4**).

9. Provide post-operative instructions; avoid eating for a minimum of 1-h.

10.2 ART restorations using HVGIC

1. Cotton wool rolls placed to isolate the tooth undergoing treatment.

2. Ensuring sufficient finger support, the tip of a sharp excavator is used to access caries.

3. During caries excavation, particular attention should be paid to removing soft dentine from Enamel-Dentine junction (EDJ).

4. In deep cavities it's acceptable to leave some soft dentine on the pulpal floor to avoid risk of pulpal exposure.

5. Once excavation has been completed, the cavity should be rinsed then dried using cotton pellets (**Figure 2-1**).

6. Condition the cavity as well as the adjacent pits and fissures using 20% polyacrylic acid.

7. Restore the cavity using properly mixed HVGIC ensuring that adjacent pits and fissures are included (**Figure 2-2**).

8. Pressure (press-finger technique) applied onto the occlusal surface using a lubricated finger for a few seconds until the GIC has initially set (**Figure 2-3**).

9. Remove finger and check that GIC has filled all occlusal surface including pits and fissures then remove excess (**Figure 2-4**).

10. Check occlusion and adjust if necessary.

11. Place a fresh layer of petroleum jelly on the occlusal surface (**Figure 2-5**).

12. Provide post-operative instructions; avoid eating for a minimum of 1-h.

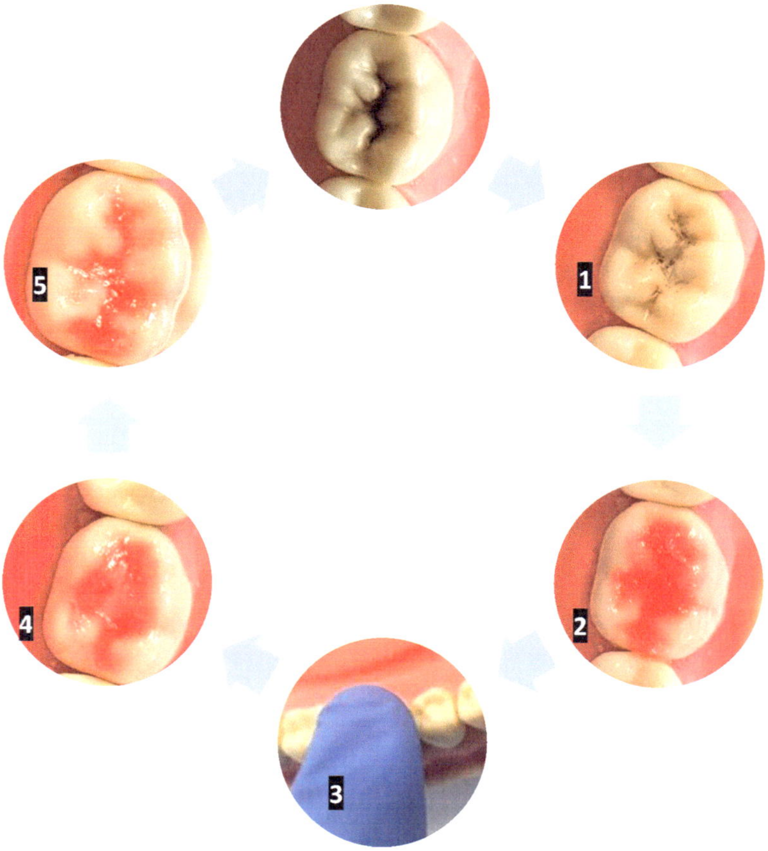

Figure 2.
Schematic representation of the steps involved in restoring cavitated teeth using HVGIC. In a clockwise direction: (1) Carious soft tissue excavated from cavity. (2) HVGIC placed in the cavity that is slightly overfilled to include the fissures. (3) Finger- press over filled cavity and adjacent pits & fissures. (5) Adjusted and finished restoration.

The above guide described ART stages for one-surface cavities. On multi-surface anterior and posterior cavities the stages are rather the same with the difference being in using the Mylar/plastic matrix strips and wedges to re-create proximal contacts.

11. Factors affecting success of ART

As previously mentioned, despite the fact that the ART is a simplified approach compared to conventional restorative treatments, restorations provided following ART can still fail or at least be compromised as a result of a break in the chain of delivering any of the procedure stages. In that, factors relating to the operator, materials used, or any breach in the technique stages could all compromise the success of ART restorations [71]. In clinical dentistry, the correct assessment to justify any treatment approach underpins the success of the treatment and therefore, ensuring suitability to perform ART on patients is of utmost importance [72]. Other operator-related factors include ensuring adequate moisture control, caries removal as recommended in the stages mentioned in the previous sections, and HVGIC handling relating to the material mixing and insertion [73]. Another aspect that has been frequently reported to have a significant impact on the success of ART restorations is the operator experience and training [74, 75]. Even in the presence of conflicting literature reports regarding the significance of moisture control, caries removal and material handling [74], there seems to be a general consensus on the importance of ART specific training in increasing the procedure success rates [36, 74–77].

The other two factors; materials and technique, have also been reported to have an impact on the long-term success of ART restorations. These are interrelated as the former relates to proper HVGIC mixing to reach the correct consistency and the latter is about soft dentine excavation, cavity conditioning and how to properly load the mixed GIC in increments into the cavity. Additionally, using the finger technique, press first then move sideways upon removal and finishing off the restoration as described in the previous research are all factors that need to be considered to ensure longevity of final restorations [37].

12. ART combination treatment

Minimal intervention dentistry is a philosophy from which other concepts for example ART have emerged. Similar conservative approaches have also been proposed with claims that the combination of which with ART could potentially result in improved ART outcomes. One of the approaches is the use of the chemo-mechanical caries removal system Carisolv™ gel (RLS Global AB, Gothenburg, Sweden) to aid in achieving caries-free cavities prior to cavity restoration [78]. Carisolv™ gel consists of a mix of sodium hypochlorite and three amino acids and its mechanism of action is through selective dentine softening to facilitate removal with hand instruments [79]. However, despite the initial promising results, it has been found that the combination of Carisolv™ gel and ART did not modify the outcomes of ART restorations [80].

Silver Diamine fluoride (SDF), originally marketed as a desensitising agent, seems to be gaining popularity for use as an adjunct to ART to prevent and arrest dental caries in both primary and permanent teeth, a procedure which is known as Silver-modified atraumatic restorative treatment (SMART) [81]. The SDF concentration of

28%, containing 44,800 ppm fluoride, has been proven to be the mostly effective in arresting dental caries [82]. In this approach, SDF is applied just before restoring with HVGIC, however, the material is notorious for leaving a permanent black stain on the arrested carious lesions which could impair aesthetics if used on anterior teeth [83]. Furthermore, research on the quality of GIC bond strength to dentine following the application of SDF has been inconsistent with few studies reported that SDF application had either no adverse effect on the adhesion of GIC to dentine [83–85] or even a significant increase in the bond strength value of GIC to dentine post SDF application [86]. On the other hand, further research in this area have demonstrated that GIC bond strength to dentine was drastically reduced following the application of SDF [87].

Further research suggested a modified form of ART, known as ARTm, when compared to the original or true ART approach [88]. The procedure involved using a high-speed diamond bur to remove unsupported enamel only while soft dentine removal to be performed using hand instruments in accordance with the original or true ART. The authors claimed that ARTm could encourage more dental practitioner to accept and adopt the ART approach, however, despite been widely used in its country of origin (Brazil), there is a need for ARTm to be recognised and approved worldwide for which further research is needed.

As a result of the above findings, it's clear that there is a huge lack of sound evidence to support the use of any of the aforementioned approaches in combination with ART and further research is needed to enable drawing evidence-based conclusions.

13. ART restorations and sealants survival rates

The outcome measures to indicate whether an ART restoration is successful or not have been reported to be either primary or secondary [89]. The primary outcomes are those where the treated tooth continued to be asymptomatic without any signs of caries progression either clinically or radiographically. The secondary outcome measures, however, indicate the failure of an ART restoration that necessitates either retreatment to remove secondary caries and the replacement of a failed or lost restoration, or performing more advanced treatment such as root canal treatment or even extraction [89].

ART restoration survival rates can be related to the simplicity of the treatment such as those involving single Vs multi-surface restorations. Generally speaking, single surface ART restorations using HVGIC showed significantly higher survival rates than those involved multi-surface cavities [36, 90]. One study has reported that after 12-months, class I and class V ART restorations showed approximately 80–90% success rates when compared to 55–75% and 35–55% for class III and class IV ART restorations, respectively [91]. Similar investigations also demonstrated that ART restorations that involved single surfaces had 95% and 97% one-year survival rates in primary and permanent teeth, respectively. Subsequently, the same restorations survival rates decreased to 86% and 72% after 3 years and 6 years, respectively [36].

ART restoration retention rates have been reported to be higher in the first year with a slight decrease in the following year with retention rates reduction from 81% to 66%, respectively [18]. Other studies have demonstrated comparable retention rates over a 3-year period which approximately ranged from 92% in the first year to 82% and 71% in the second & third years, respectively [92]. In general, there seems to be an increased research to support that HVGIC ART restorations have either comparable or longer survival rates than conventional restorative treatments and composite restorations [90, 92].

ART sealant survival rates on the other hand were assessed based on whether sealants have been either partially or completely dislodged over a period of three years [36]. At the one- and three-year follow-up research, HVGIC ART sealants were found to have had higher survival rates compared to using low- or medium viscosity GIC and the resin-based sealants when performed under the same application conditions [36, 93]. The above survival rates provided research evidence to further support the effectiveness of ART approach in the management of dental caries.

14. To repair or to replace failed ART restorations

When indicated, repairing defective ART restoration remains the preferred approach to replacing the whole restoration [94]. It has been stated that replacing restorations involves the likelihood of further tooth tissue loss that despite being minimal, the increased number of interventions could increase the amount of tissue loss [95]. Also, from an experience perspective, it has been reported that patients tended to have less levels of anxiety when restoration repair was planned [95].

All initial carious lesions can successfully be treated following the minimally intervention approach [96]. A new approach to define carious lesions has been devised as a guide to facilitate identification of the lesions based on their site and size [97]. ART restoration failures can vary from material wear of more than 0.5 mm, partial or complete material loss or caries around cavity margins, the management of which again varies from material top up to cavity cleaning and conditioning or complete material replacement [72].

This has placed further emphasis on the 'means to prevent failure' to avoid the need for repairing or replacing ART restorations starting with an accurate decision regarding the suitability of teeth to receive ART and when restoration failure exists to perform a vigilant tooth and restoration assessment to identify the failure and its best management approach.

15. ART and the Covid-19 pandemic era

Since its outbreak, Covid-19 has caused disruption to the provision of dental treatments with new guidelines released in response to regulate treatment delivery without compromising safety standards [98, 99]. As a result of the pandemic restrictions and the subsequent changes in providing routine dentistry non-aerosol generating procedures (non-AGPs) where the use of minimally or non-invasive instead of the conventional treatment approaches were highly recommended [97]. There have been a few reports indicating that using ART during the pandemic would have been successful given all the positive outcomes reported in the literature [100, 101]. Furthermore, as it does not involve the use of rotary instruments, ART is not considered an AGP and therefore requires no fallow times [102] which are known to may have an impact on the capacity for providing dental care.

Despite the fact that restrictions have eased, the Covid-19 virus and its variants are still present and every precaution should be taken to prevent the risk of the disease transmission by avoiding elective AGPs and using minimally or non-invasive approaches such as ART. Nonetheless, making appropriate clinical decisions alongside integrating prevention-centred practices should remain a cornerstone to use in adjunct to ART approach as part of embracing all minimally invasive caries management strategies.

16. Conclusion

Despite the increased focus within dental institutes in the UK and other developed countries to teach and encourage students to perform minimally invasive caries management, true ART has not gained similar popularity particularly among primary care dental practitioners. Furthermore, and in spite of the existing evidence regarding ART effectiveness as a minimally invasive caries management approach there is still a distinct lack of research regarding the perception and practice of ART in primary care settings. Operator experience remains a significant factor in achieving higher ART success rates particularly when combined with specific ART training to enhance skills to achieve best results. ART success is also dependent on careful consideration of other factors such as patient and tooth assessment to ensure suitability to receive ART with a clear emphasis on repairing failed restorations when clinically indicated rather than replacement.

Another significant aspect of the ART concept is its role in the prevention promotion programme that accompanies the restorative care. In that, an oral health care plan in the form of caries assessment and education regarding tailored prevention strategies should be determined and discussed with patients. Those should continuously be assessed and reinforced during the appropriate review appointments.

It is apparent that ART can be the alternative caries prevention and treatment approach of choice particularly in the current continuing Covid-19 era. Even with the easing pandemic restrictions, practising safe dentistry is still of paramount importance further indicating that true ART and possibly its modified forms, ARTm and SMART, would have a great potential to be appropriate caries treatment strategies and could therefore become the old-new normal caries management approaches.

Acknowledgements

The author would like to thank the University of Liverpool for supporting the publication of this chapter through completely covering the required funds.

Conflict of interest

The author declares no conflict of interest.

Author details

Manal A. Ablal
School of Dentistry, Institute of Life Course and Medical Sciences, The University of Liverpool, Liverpool, United Kingdom

*Address all correspondence to: maaablal@liverpool.ac.uk

References

[1] Pitts NB, Zero DT, Marsh PD, Ekstrand K, Weintraub JA, Ramos-Gomez F, et al. Dental caries. Nature Reviews Disease Primers. 2017;**25**(3):17030. DOI: 10.1038/nrdp.2017.30

[2] Chen X, Daliri EB, Tyagi A, Oh DH. Cariogenic biofilm: Pathology-related phenotypes and targeted therapy. Microorganisms. 2021;**9**(6):1311. DOI: 10.3390/microorganisms9061311

[3] Jodłowska A, Leś-Smolarczyk A, Postek-Stefańska L. Description of five deep caries management methods and their use in contemporary dentistry. Journal of Stomatology. 2018;**71**(3):3 02-307. DOI: 10.5114/jos.2018.80639

[4] Armfield JM, Heaton LJ. Management of fear and anxiety in the dental clinic: A review. Australian Dental Journal. 2013;**58**(4):390-407; quiz 531. DOI: 10.1111/adj.12118

[5] University of Sydney [Internet]. 2015. 'No-drill' Dentistry Stops Tooth Decay. Science Daily. Available from: www.sciencedaily.com/releases/2015/12/151206164802.htm. [Accessed: April 01, 2022]

[6] Global, regional, and national incidence, prevalence, and years lived with disability for 354 diseases and injuries for 195 countries and territories, 1990-2017: Systematic analysis for the Global Burden of Disease Study 2017. Lancet. 2018;**392**(10159):1789-1858

[7] Croll TP, Berg J. Delivery of fluoride solutions to proximal tooth surfaces. Part II: Caries interception with silver diamine fluoride. Inside Dentistry. 2017;**13**(9):56-58

[8] Frencken JE, Peters MC, Manton DJ, Leal SC, Gordan VV, Eden E. Minimal intervention dentistry for managing dental caries—A review: Report of a FDI task group. International Dental Journal. 2012;**62**(5):223-243. DOI: 10.1111/idj.12007

[9] Walsh LJ, Brostek AM. Minimum intervention dentistry principles and objectives. Australian Dental Journal. 2013;**58**(Suppl. 1):3-16. DOI: 10.1111/adj.12045

[10] Horowitz AM. Introduction to the symposium on minimal intervention techniques for caries. Journal of Public Health Dentistry. 1996;**56**(3 Spec):133-134; discussion 161-3. DOI: 10.1111/j.1752-7325.1996.tb02422.x

[11] Tyas MJ, Anusavice KJ, Frencken JE, Mount GJ. Minimal intervention dentistry—A review. FDI Commission Project 1-97. International Dental Journal. 2000;**50**(1):1-12. DOI: 10.1111/j.1875-595x.2000.tb00540.x

[12] Saber AM, El-Housseiny AA, Alamoudi NM. Atraumatic restorative treatment and interim therapeutic restoration: A review of the literature. Dentistry Journal (Basel). 2019;**7**(1):28. DOI: 10.3390/dj7010028

[13] Leal SC, Abreu DM, Frencken JE. Dental anxiety and pain related to ART. Journal of Applied Oral Science. 2009;**17**:84-88. DOI: 10.1590/s1678-77572009000700015

[14] Garg Y, Bhaskar DJ, Suvarna M, Singh N, Lata S, Bose S. Atraumatic restorative treatment in dentistry. International Journal of Oral Health and Medical Research. 2015;**2**(2):126-129

[15] Frencken JE, Makoni F, Sithole WD, Hackenitz E. Three-year survival of

one-surface ART restorations and glass-ionomer sealants in a school oral health programme in Zimbabwe. Caries Research. 1998;**32**(2):119-126. DOI: 10.1159/000016441

[16] Holmgren CJ, Roux D, Doméjean S. Minimal intervention dentistry: Part 5. Atraumatic restorative treatment (ART)-a minimum intervention and minimally invasive approach for the management of dental caries. British Dental Journal. 2013;**214**(1):11-18. DOI: 10.1038/sj.bdj.2012.1175

[17] Molina GF, Faulks D, Frencken J. Acceptability, feasibility and perceived satisfaction of the use of the atraumatic restorative treatment approach for people with disability. Brazilian Oral Research. 2015;**29**:S1806. DOI: 10.1590/1807-3107BOR-2015.vol29.0097

[18] Indications of ART, Sharma S, Raghu R, Shetty A. Current status of atraumatic restorative treatment in restorative dentistry. Journal of Restorative Dentistry and Endodontics. 2021;**1**(1):9-16. DOI: 10.25259/JRDE_8_2020

[19] Lopez N, Simpser-Rafalin S, Berthold P. Atraumatic restorative treatment for prevention and treatment of caries in an underserved community. American Journal of Public Health. 2005;**95**(8):1338-1339. DOI: 10.2105/AJPH.2004.056945

[20] Farag A, Frencken JE. Acceptance and discomfort from atraumatic restorative treatment in secondary school students in Egypt. Medical Principles and Practice. 2009;**18**(1):26-30. DOI: 10.1159/000163042

[21] Kikwilu EN, Frencken J, Mulder J. Impact of Atraumatic Restorative Treatment (ART) on the treatment profile in pilot government dental clinics in Tanzania. BMC Oral Health. 2009;**8**(9):14. DOI: 10.1186/1472-6831-9-14

[22] Cole BO, Welbury RR. The atraumatic restorative treatment (ART) technique: Does it have a place in everyday practice? Dental Update. 2000;**27**(3):118-120, 122-3. DOI: 10.12968/denu.2000.27.3.118

[23] Burke FJ, McHugh S, Shaw L, Hosey MT, Macpherson L, Delargy S, et al. UK dentists' attitudes and behaviour towards atraumatic restorative treatment for primary teeth. British Dental Journal. 2005;**199**(6):365-369; discussion 353; quiz 372. DOI: 10.1038/sj.bdj.4812696

[24] Fusayama T, Terachima S. Differentiation of two layers of carious dentin by staining. Journal of Dental Research. 1972;**51**(3):866

[25] Schwendicke F, Innes N. Removal strategies for carious tissues in deep lesions. In: Schwendicke F, editor. Management of Deep Carious Lesions. Cham: Springer; 2018. DOI: https://doi-org.liverpool.idm.oclc.org/10.1007/978-3-319-61370-3_2

[26] Kidd E, Fejerskov O, Nyvad B. Infected dentine revisited. Dental Update. 2015, 2015;**42**(9):802-806; 808-9. DOI: 10.12968/denu.2015.42.9.802

[27] Banerjee A. Selective removal of carious dentin. In: Schwendicke F, editor. Management of Deep Carious Lesions. Cham: Springer; 2018. DOI: https://doi-org.liverpool.idm.oclc.org/10.1007/978-3-319-61370-3_5

[28] Farges JC, Alliot-Licht B, Renard E, Ducret M, Gaudin A, Smith AJ, et al. Dental pulp defence and repair mechanisms in dental caries. Mediators of Inflammation. 2015;**230251**. DOI: 10.1155/2015/230251

[29] Schwendicke F, Frencken JE, Bjørndal L, Maltz M, Manton DJ, Ricketts D, et al. Managing carious lesions: Consensus recommendations on carious tissue removal. Advances in Dental Research. 2016;**28**(2):58-67. DOI: 10.1177/0022034516639271

[30] Frencken JE, Leal SC, Navarro MF. Twenty-five-year atraumatic restorative treatment (ART) approach: A comprehensive overview. Clinical Oral Investigations. 2012;**16**(5):1337-1346. DOI: 10.1007/s00784-012-0783-4

[31] Erickson RL, Glasspoole EA. Bonding to tooth structure: A comparison of glass ionomer and composite-resin systems. Journal of Esthetic Dentistry. 1994;**6**: 227-244. DOI: 10.1111/j.1708-8240.1994.tb00864.x

[32] Swartz ML, Phillips RW, Clark HE. Long-term F release from glass ionomer cements. Journal of Dental Research. 1984;**63**(2):158-160. DOI: 10.1177/00220345840630021301

[33] Forsten L. Fluoride release and uptake by glass-ionomers and related materials and its clinical effect. Biomaterials. 1998;**19**(6):503-508. DOI: 10.1016/s0142-9612(97)00130-0

[34] Leyhausen G, Abtahi M, Karbakhsch M, Sapotnick A, Geurtsen W. Biocompatibility of various light-curing and one conventional glass-ionomer cement. Biomaterials. 1998;**19**:559-564. DOI: 10.1016/s0142-9612(97)00137-3

[35] Bullard RH, Leinfelder KF, Russell CM. Effect of coefficient of thermal expansion on microleakage. Journal of American Dental Association. 1998;**116**:871-874. DOI: 10.14219/jada.archive.1988.0291

[36] van't Hof MA, Frencken JE, van Palenstein Helderman WH, Holmgren CJ. The atraumatic restorative treatment (ART) approach for managing dental caries: A meta-analysis. International Dental Journal. 2006;**56**(6):345-351. DOI: 10.1111/j.1875-595x.2006.tb00339.x

[37] Frencken JE. The state-of-the-ART of ART sealants. Dental Update. 2014;**41**(2):119-120, 122-4. DOI: 10.12968/denu.2014.41.2.119

[38] Bonifácio CC, Kleverlaan CJ, Raggio DP, Werner A, de Carvalho RC, van Amerongen WE. Physical-mechanical properties of glass ionomer cements indicated for atraumatic restorative treatment. Australian Dental Journal. 2009;**54**(3):233-237. DOI: 10.1111/j.1834-7819.2009. 01125.x

[39] Shivanna MM, Ganesh S, Khanagar SB, Naik S, Divakar DD, Al-Kheraif AA, et al. Twelve-month evaluation of the atraumatic restorative treatment approach for class III restorations: An interventional study. World Journal of Clinical Cases. 2020;**8**(18):3999-4009. DOI: 10.12998/wjcc.v8.i18.3999

[40] Brostek AM, Bochenek AJ, Walsh LJ. Minimally invasive dentistry: A review and update. Shanghai Kou Qiang Yi Xue. 2006;**15**(3):225-249

[41] Mandari GJ, Frencken JE, van't Hof MA. Six-year success rates of occlusal amalgam and glass-ionomer restorations placed using three minimal intervention approaches. Caries Research. 2003;**37**(4):246-253. DOI: 10.1159/000070866

[42] Bali P, Prabhakar AR, Basappa N. An in vitro comparative evaluation of compressive strength and antibacterial activity of conventional GIC and hydroxyapatite reinforced GIC in different storage media. Journal of Clinical and Diagnostic Research.

2015;**9**(7):ZC51-ZC55. DOI: 10.7860/JCDR/2015/13012.6205

[43] Yilmaz Y, Eyuboglu O, Kocogullari ME, Belduz N. A one-year clinical evaluation of a high-viscosity glass ionomer cement in primary molars. Journal of Contemporary Dental Practice. 2006;**7**(1):71-78

[44] Phonghanyudh A, Theerareungchaisri C, Jirarattanasopa V. Clinical evaluation of class II high-viscosity glass ionomer cement and composite resin restorations in primary molars: One-year result. Mahidol Dental Journal. 2014;**34**(2):129-136

[45] van Duinen RN, Kleverlaan CJ, de Gee AJ, Werner A, Feilzer AJ. Early and long-term wear of 'fast-set' conventional glass-ionomer cements. Dental Materials. 2005;**21**(8):716-720. DOI: 10.1016/j.dental.2004.09.007

[46] Dülgergil CT, Soyman M, Civelek A. Atraumatic restorative treatment with resin-modified glass ionomer material: Short-term results of a pilot study. Medical Principles and Practice. 2005;**14**(4):277-280. DOI: 10.1159/000085750

[47] de Souza EM, Cefaly DF, Terada RS, Rodrigues CC, de Lima Navarro MF. Clinical evaluation of the ART technique using high density and resin-modified glass lonomer cements. Oral Health and Preventive Dentistry. 2003;**1**(3):201-207

[48] Ercan E, Dülgergil CT, Soyman M, Dalli M, Yildirim I. A field-trial of two restorative materials used with atraumatic restorative treatment in rural Turkey: 24-month results. Journal of Applied Oral Science. 2009;**17**(4):307-314. DOI: 10.1590/s1678-77572009000400008

[49] Berzins DW, Abey S, Costache MC, Wilkie CA, Roberts HW. Resin-modified glass-ionomer setting reaction competition. Journal of Dental Research. 2010;**89**(1):82-86. DOI: 10.1177/0022034509355919

[50] Rodrigues MP, Cunha LSD, Vilela ABF, Schettini ACT, Bragança GF, França R, et al. Selective carious tissue removal and glass ionomer liner reduction of pulp stress in bulk fill resin composite restorations. Brazilian Oral Research. 2021;**35**:e119. DOI: 10.1590/1807-3107bor-2021.vol35.0119

[51] Berg JH. The continuum of restorative materials in pediatric dentistry—A review for the clinician. Pediatric Dentistry. 1998;**20**(2):93-100

[52] Medeiros FD, Santos MM, Araújo IJ, Lima IP. Clinical evaluation of two materials in the restoration of abfraction lesions. Brazilian Journal of Oral Sciences. 2015;**14**:287-293. DOI: 10.1590/1677-3225v14n4a07

[53] Frencken JE. Atraumatic restorative treatment and minimal intervention dentistry. British Dental Journal. 2017;**223**(3):183-189. DOI: 10.1038/sj.bdj.2017.664

[54] Jackson RD. New posterior composite materials improving placement efficiency. Compendium of Continuing Education in Dentistry. 2012;**33**(4):292-293

[55] Tsujimoto A, Barkmeier WW, Takamizawa T, Latta MA, Miyazaki M. Mechanical properties, volumetric shrinkage and depth of cure of short fiber-reinforced resin composite. Dental Materials Journal. 2016;**35**(3):418-424. DOI: 10.4012/dmj.2015-280

[56] Soares CJ, Faria-E-Silva AL, Rodrigues MP, Vilela ABF, Pfeifer CS, Tantbirojn, et al. Polymerization

shrinkage stress of composite resins and resin cements: What do we need to know? Brazilian Oral Research. 2017;**31**(Suppl. 1): 0062. DOI: 10.1590/1807-3107BOR-2017. vol31.0062

[57] Ehlers V, Gran K, Callaway A, Azrak B, Ernst CP. One-year clinical performance of flowable bulk-fill composite vs conventional compomer restorations in primary molars. Journal of Adhesive Dentistry. 2019;**21**(3):247-254. DOI: 10.3290/j.jad.a42519

[58] Louw AJ, Sarvan I, Chikte UM, Honkala E. One-year evaluation of atraumatic restorative treatment and minimum intervention techniques on primary teeth. South African Dental Journal. 2002;**57**(9):366-371

[59] Olegário IC, Hesse D, Mendes FM, Bonifácio CC, Raggio DP. Glass carbomer and compomer for ART restorations: 3-year results of a randomized clinical trial. Clinical Oral Investigations. 2019;**23**(4):1761-1770. DOI: 10.1007/s00784-018-2593-9

[60] Gerdolle DA, Mortier E, Droz D. Microleakage and polymerization shrinkage of various polymer restorative materials. Journal of Dentistry for Children (Chic). 2008;**75**(2):125-133

[61] Frencken JE. Evolution of the the ART approach: Highlights and achievements. Journal of Applied Oral Science. 2009;**17**(Suppl(spe)):78-83. DOI: 10.1590/s1678-77572009000700014

[62] Frencken JE, Pilot T, Songpaisan Y, Phantumvanit P. Atraumatic restorative treatment (ART): Rationale, technique and development. Journal of Public Health Dentistry. 1996;**56**:135-140. DOI: 10.1111/j.1752-7325. 1996.tb02423.x

[63] Frencken JE, van Amerongen WE. The Atraumatic restorative treatment approach. In: Fejerskov O, Kidd E, editors. Dental Caries: The Disease and its Clinical Management. 2nd ed. Oxford: Blackwell Munksgaard; 2008. pp. 427-442

[64] Naaman R, El-Housseiny AA, Alamoudi N. The use of pit and fissure sealants—A literature review. Dentistry Journal (Basel). 2017;**5**(4):34. DOI: 10.3390/dj5040034

[65] Sreedevi A, Brizuela M, Mohamed S. Pit and fissure sealants. In: StatPearls [Internet]. Treasure Island (FL): StatPearls Publishing; 2021

[66] WHO Oral Health Programme. Atraumatic Restorative Treatment (ART) for Tooth Decay: A Global Initiative 1998-2000. World Health Organisation. Available from: https://apps.who.int/iris/handle/10665/64325

[67] Frencken J, Frencken J, WHO Collaborating Centre for Oral Health Services Research. Manual for the Atraumatic Restorative Treatment Approach to Control Dental Caries. Groningen, The Netherlands: WHO Collaborating Centre for Oral Health Services Research; 1997

[68] da Mata C, McKenna G, Anweigi L, Hayes M, Cronin M, Woods N, et al. An RCT of atraumatic restorative treatment for older adults: 5-year results. Journal of Dentistry. 2009;**83**:95-99. DOI: 10.1016/j.jdent.2019.03.003

[69] Nkwocha FG, Akinyamoju CA, Ogbode SO, Lawal FB. Management of dental caries with atraumatic restorative treatment under field condition in primary schools in oyo state, Nigeria. Annals of Ibadan Postgraduate Medicine. 2019;**17**(1):75-80. Erratum in: Annals of Ibadan Postgraduate Medicine. 2019;17(2):203

[70] Breslin, M., Cook S. No turning back: Posture in dental practice (2015). BDJ Team 2, 15164. 10.1038/bdjteam.2015.164

[71] Mickenautsch S, Grossman E. Atraumatic restorative treatment (ART): Factors affecting success. Journal of Applied Oral Science. 2006;**14**(Suppl):34-36. DOI: 10.1590/s1678-77572006000700008

[72] Karthavya S. Atraumatic Restorative Treatment. International Journal of Science and Research (IJSR). 2017;**6**(8):1095-1097

[73] da Franca C, Colares V, Van Amerongen E. The operator as a factor of success in ART restorations. Brazilian Journal of Oral Sciences. 2011;**10**(1):60-64. DOI: 10.20396/bjos.v10i1.8641699

[74] Jiang M, Fan Y, Li KY, Lo ECM, Chu CH, Wong MCM. Factors affecting success rate of atraumatic restorative treatment (ART) restorations in children: A systematic review and meta-analysis. Journal of Dentistry. 2021;**104**:103526. DOI: 10.1016/j.jdent.2020.103526

[75] Luengas-Quintero E, Frencken JE, Muñúzuri-Hernández JA, Mulder J. The atraumatic restorative treatment (ART) strategy in Mexico: Two-years follow up of ART sealants and restorations. BMC Oral Health. 2013;**13**:42. DOI: 10.1186/1472-6831-13-42

[76] Frencken JE, Leal SC. The correct use of the ART approach. Journal of Applied Oral Science. 2010;**18**(1):1-4. DOI: 10.1590/s1678-77572010000100002

[77] Molina G, Kultje C. Atraumatic restorative treatment with Carisolv (TM) in mentally disabled patients. Journal of Dental Research. 2001;**80**(4):963-963

[78] Kirzioglu Z, Gurbuz T, Yilmaz Y. Clinical evaluation of chemomechanical and mechanical caries removal: Status of the restorations at 3, 6, 9 and 12 months. Clinical Oral Investigations. 2007;**11**(1):69-76. DOI: 10.1007/s00784-006-0072-1

[79] Gil-Montoya JA, Mateos-Palacios R, Bravo M, González-Moles MA, Pulgar R. Atraumatic restorative treatment and Carisolv use for root caries in the elderly: 2-year follow-up randomized clinical trial. Clinical Oral Investigations. 2014;**18**(4):1089-1095. DOI: 10.1007/s00784-013-1087-z

[80] Seifo N, Cassie H, Radford JR, Innes NPT. Silver diamine fluoride for managing carious lesions: An umbrella review. BMC Oral Health. 2019;**19**(1):145. DOI: 10.1186/s12903-019-0830-5

[81] Seifo N, Robertson M, MacLean J, Blain K, Grosse S, Milne R, et al. The use of silver diamine fluoride (SDF) in dental practice. British Dental Journal. 2020;**228**(2):75-81. DOI: 10.1038/s41415-020-1203-9

[82] Jiang M, Mei ML, Wong MCM, Chu CH, Lo ECM. Effect of silver diamine fluoride solution application on the bond strength of dentine to adhesives and to glass ionomer cements: A systematic review. BMC Oral Health. 2020;**20**(1):40. DOI: 10.1186/s12903-020-1030-z

[83] Puwanawiroj A, Trairatvorakul C, Dasanayake AP, Auychai P. Microtensile bond strength between glass ionomer cement and silver diamine fluoride-treated carious primary dentin. Pediatric Dentistry. 2018;**40**(4):291-295

[84] Zhao IS, Chu S, Yu OY, Mei ML, Chu CH, Lo ECM. Effect of silver diamine fluoride and potassium iodide on shear bond strength of glass ionomer cements to caries-affected dentine. International Dental Journal. 2019;**69**(5):341-347. DOI: 10.1111/idj.12478

[85] Gupta J, Thomas MS, Radhakrishna M, Srikant N, Ginjupalli K. Effect of silver diamine fluoride-potassium iodide and 2% chlorhexidine gluconate cavity cleansers on the bond strength and microleakage of resin-modified glass ionomer cement. Journal of Conservative Dentistry. 2019;**22**(2):201-206. DOI: 10.4103/JCD.JCD_485_18

[86] Knight GM, McIntyre JM, Mulyani. The effect of silver fluoride and potassium iodide on the bond strength of auto cure glass ionomer cement to dentine. Australian Dental Journal. 2006;**51**(1):42-45. DOI: 10.1111/j.1834-7819. 2006.tb00399.x

[87] Massara Mde L, Bönecker M. Modified ART: Why not? Brazilian Oral Research. 2012;**26**(3):187-189. DOI: 10.1590/s1806-83242012000300001

[88] BaniHani A, Santamaría RM, Hu S, Maden M, Albadri S. Minimal intervention dentistry for managing carious lesions into dentine in primary teeth: An umbrella review. European Archives of Paediatric Dentistry. 2021 [Accessed April 10, 2022]. DOI: 10.1007/s40368-021-00675-6

[89] Molina GF, Faulks D, Mulder J, Frencken JE. High-viscosity glass-ionomer vs. composite resin restorations in persons with disability: Five-year follow-up of clinical trial. Brazilian Oral Research. 2019;**33**:e099. DOI: 10.1590/1807-3107bor-2019.vol33.0099

[90] Smales RJ, Yip HK. The atraumatic restorative treatment (ART) approach for primary teeth: Review of literature. Pediatric Dentistry. 2000;**22**(4):294-298

[91] Mjör IA, Gordan VV. A review of atraumatic restorative treatment (ART). International Dental Journal. 1999;**49**(3):127-131. DOI: 10.1002/j.1875-595x.1999.tb00896.x

[92] de Amorim RG, Leal SC, Frencken JE. Survival of atraumatic restorative treatment (ART) sealants and restorations: A meta-analysis. Clinical Oral Investigations. 2012;**16**(2):429-441. DOI: 10.1007/s00784-011-0513-3

[93] Goldberg M. Atraumatic restorative treatment (ART). JSM Dentistry. 2020;**8**(2):1126

[94] Javidi H, Tickle M, Aggarwal VR. Repair vs replacement of failed restorations in general dental practice: Factors influencing treatment choices and outcomes. British Dental Journal. 2015;**218**(1):E2. DOI: 10.1038/sj.bdj.2014.1165

[95] Mount GJ, Ngo H. Minimal intervention: Early lesions. Quintessence International. 2000;**31**(8):535-546

[96] Mount GJ, Hume WR. A new cavity classification. Australian Dental Journal. 1998;**43**(3):153-159. DOI: 10.1111/j.1834-7819. 1998.tb00156.x

[97] British Endodontic Society. BES COVID-19 Return to Work SOP [Internet]. 2021. Available from: https://britishendodonticsociety.org.uk/wp-content/uploads/2021/12/BES_SOP_1.5.pdf. [Accessed: April 01, 2022]

[98] Scottish Dental Clinical Effectiveness Programme. Mitigation of Aerosol Generating Procedures in Dentistry. Report on Recent Published Evidence [Internet]. 2021. Available from: https://www.sdcep.org.uk/wp-content/uploads/2021/04/SDCEP-Report-on-Recent-PublishedEvidence-April-2021.pdf. [Accessed: April 01, 2022]

[99] Al-Halabi M, Salami A, Alnuaimi E, Kowash M, Hussein I. Assessment of paediatric dental guidelines and caries management alternatives in the post

COVID-19 period. A critical review and clinical recommendations. European Archives of Paediatric Dentistry. 2020;**21**(5):543-556. DOI: 10.1007/s40368-020-00547-5

[100] Nandlal B, Singh B, Gopi A. Impact on utilization and shift in treatment needs post-COVID lockdown of pediatric dentistry in a tertiary care hospital. Frontiers in Dental Medicine. 2021;**2**:722292. DOI: 10.3389/fdmed.2021.722292

[101] Maru V. The 'new normal' in post-COVID-19 pediatric dental practice. International Journal of Paediatric Dentistry. 2021;**31**(4):528-538. DOI: 10.1111/ipd.12764

[102] Bahia G, Janjua U, Ashfaq N. Atraumatic restorative technique & its role in the COVID-19 pandemic. The Dentist. 2021;**2**(1):1017

Chapter 7

The Frequency of Different Liners Usages in Upper and Lower Anterior Teeth at Dentistry Teaching Clinic Patients in Kabul, Afghanistan

Husniya Azim and Shiba Azim

Abstract

The use of liners to maintain the vitality and health of dental pulp is an effective method in operative dentistry, which involves placing a protective layer of liner on the exposed pulp to maintain the health of pulp and stimulate dentin cells to make reparative dentin. The use of liners for pulp vitality has been used for many years and is considered an essential part of restorative procedures in operative dentistry textbooks. Liners have traditionally been used to protect the pulp from the potentially toxic effects of different irritants. Liners are currently used for their therapeutic effects or for sealing dentinal tubules against the penetration of microorganisms or their by-products. Different types of materials have been introduced as liners to protect pulp tissue from irritants. Liner materials that have been used for many years include calcium hydroxide, glass-ionomer, and modified resin glass-ionomer. Therefore, this study, performed in the Dentistry Teaching Clinic of Kabul, Afghanistan, aims to present the most frequently clinically used liners in anterior teeth, to maintain pulp vitality.

Keywords: liners, calcium hydroxide, zinc oxide eugenol, glass ionomer, mineral trioxide aggregate

1. Introduction

One of the main goals of operative dentistry is to protect the health of dental pulp, which can be provided by using liners. Liners are materials that have the healing ability and sealing properties of dentinal tubules, protect the pulp from chemical, mechanical, and thermal stimuli and stimulate the formation of reparative dentin. Liners are used as a specific thickness in preparing cavities on the pulp to maintain the pulp health. In the anterior teeth, the use of liners has particular importance to protect the dental pulp [1].

In this study, the different usage of liner in the anterior maxillary and mandibular teeth to preserve the pulp and prevent tooth extraction to evaluate the effectiveness of each liner in the future to obtain better clinical results.

The volume of the anterior teeth is smaller than the posterior teeth according to anatomical structure, and if there is caries or any defect that requires a dental filling, the size of the prepared cavity is small or with a preparing cavity, each cavity walls may near contact to the dental pulp or pulp horn. So, in such cases, the use of liners is mandatory and requires special technical care in the clinical procedure so that a certain size of the liner is placed in the cavity and the space prepared for permanent filling materials is not occupied by the liner to interfere with retention and resistance form of the cavity [1].

A study by Naji Ziad Arandi, in 2017, suggested that one of the goals of operative dentistry is, to maintain the health of the pulp in teeth with caries and defects. For the mentioned goal, liners are placed in a certain size in preparing cavities for maintaining the health of the pulp which is exposed or not exposed and stimulating the reparative dentin to make new dentin. The use of pulp preservative liners has been practiced in the field of dentistry for many years and is still considered an essential part of restorative procedures in operative dentistry textbooks [2].

Liners have previously been used to protect pulp tissue from the potentially toxic effects of different irritants. Currently, liners are used to treat and seal the dentinal tubules against the penetration of microorganisms or their toxic products into the teeth. Different liners introduced to protect pulp tissue from stimuli include Mineral Trioxide Aggregate (MTA), calcium hydroxide, Glass Ionomer (GI), Zinc Oxide Eugenol (ZOE), Modified Resin Glass-Ionomer (MRGI), and flowable composites [3].

Several liners have been proposed to protect the pulp. Interestingly, none of them has a significant advantage among doctors. In a survey of doctors, what kind of liners do they use, respondents mentioned four different substances, none of which are preferred by the majority of users [4].

Zinc oxide eugenol has been used in the dental sector for many years as a base, liner, cement, and temporary filling materials. Its use for direct pulp capping is questionable because the eugenol in its composition, is highly cytotoxic and shows ZOE interfacial leakage, but this leakage is not debatable because the eugenol released seals this leakage biologically and reduces bacteria [4].

A human clinical study using ZOE as a direct pulp capping agent showed in all teeth treated with ZOE as a liner, chronic pulp inflammation, without improving pulp tissue, and dentin bridge formation up to 12 weeks after the procedure was shown. Conversely, all control teeth lined with calcium hydroxide showed improvement within 4 weeks [4].

Glass Ionomer and Resin-Modified Glass Ionomer are not as cytotoxic as ZOE but become cytotoxic when in direct contact with cells. GI is less toxic than RMGI, but it is still not a good choice for pulp protection in deep cavities. GI binds chemically to the tooth structure to prevent the penetration of potentially toxic substances through the dentin into the pulp. Glass ionomer prevents bacteria to penetrate the pulp and has biocompatible properties but should not be in contact with pulp tissue. Direct pulp capping with RMGI showed chronic inflammation and no dentin bridge formation up to 300 days after the procedure, while calcium hydroxide control groups showed significantly better pulp healing [4].

Calcium hydroxide was introduced in the field of dentistry in 1921 and has been considered a direct pulp cap material for several decades as the "gold standard." There are several benefits of calcium hydroxide known as the gold standard. Calcium hydroxide has excellent antibacterial properties, and a study showed a 100% reduction in microorganisms associated with pulp infection after 1 hour of exposure to calcium hydroxide. Most importantly, calcium hydroxide has a long history of clinical success as a direct pulp cap agent for up to 10 years. Calcium hydroxide also has some disadvantages. Its self-cure form is very soluble and dissolves over time. However, it has been noted that the formation of the dentin bridge occurs until calcium hydroxide is lost due to dissolution. Calcium hydroxide does not have adhesive properties and has poor sealing power. Another critique of calcium hydroxide is the term "tunnel defects" in reparative dentin, which forms under the pulp cap. The tunnel defect is described as a pathway from the pulp exposure and through reparative dentin to the pulp. Sometimes fibroblasts and capillaries are present inside the tunnel defect. Other researchers have found that the quality of reparative dentin improves with the thickening of the dentin bridge so that many cases of tunnel defects do not remain as a communication path to the pulp. Tunnel defect does not appear to be a common finding in human studies involving direct pulp capping with calcium hydroxide. There are fewer studies that indicate the existence of a tunnel defect and there are more studies that have not reported a tunnel defect [5, 6].

Calcium hydroxide is believed to have one or more mechanisms of action on the restorative effects of the pulp tissue. Calcium hydroxide has antibacterial properties and can minimize or eliminate bacterial infiltration into the pulp. It was previously believed that the high pH of calcium hydroxide stimulated pulp tissue, which in turn slowed down the healing process through some unknown mechanism. In recent years, this "unknown mechanism" has been explained by the release of bioactive molecules that combine different types of proteins with dentin matrix during dentinogenesis. At least two of these proteins, Bone Morphogenic Protein and Transforming Growth Factor-Beta One (TBF-β1), are important in the pulp cap process because they can stimulate pulp repair. Calcium hydroxide dissolves these proteins from dentin and, upon release of these bioactive molecules, acts as a significant mediator in pulp repair after pulp capping [6].

In recent years, MTA has been introduced as pulp cap material, which shows a significant interest of doctors in this new material. MTA consists of calcium oxide in the form of tricalcium silicate, dicalcium silicate, and tricalcium aluminate to which bismuth oxide has been added for radiopaque. MTA is compatible with tissues. Interestingly, the product of the initial reaction of MTA with water is calcium hydroxide, which the formation of calcium hydroxide provides the ability to be compatible with tissue in MTA. As a result, many of the potential benefits and mechanisms of action for MTA are similar to those of calcium hydroxide, including antibacterial properties, tissue compatibility properties, high pH, radiopaque, and the ability to release dentin bioactive proteins. There are differences between MTA and calcium hydroxide. First, MTA is available in two colors, white and gray, with a gray version due to the addition of iron. Another notable difference is that MTA provides the ability to seal tooth structures well. There are also several disadvantages of MTA, including its high solubility and 24% loss after 78 days of storage in water. The presence of iron in its gray form may indicate a darker tooth color. One of the significant disadvantages of MTA is its long-term hardening of about 2 hours and 45 minutes, which requires pulp capping with MTA in two stages, so placing a temporary filling on top of the MTA before placing a permanent filling or using a fast-hardening liner is essential to protect the MTA before permanent filling. The price of 1 gram of MTA powder is approximately 24 grams of calcium hydroxide, which can be considered one of its disadvantages [6].

In a review of animal pulp capping studies comparing MTA with calcium hydroxide, general improvement of pulp with MTA was generally reported. However, in most human studies, similar results have been shown with pulp capping as a result of the use of MTA and calcium hydroxide. Among the studies, only two showed superior performance of MTA over calcium hydroxide because MTA has a better ability to seal the exposed area of the pulp than calcium hydroxide. Studies show that MTA, as the only pulp-cap material without a control group, has shown success over periods of 6 months to 4 years [6].

Different theories are available when using liners. A study conducted by R. Weiner in 2011 at a dental school in North America did not agree on the use and timing of liners. In an amalgam-filled deep cavity, 46 percent of the 52 schools of dentistry supported the use of glass ionomer as a liner. This study considers cavities with 1 mm remaining dentin thickness as deep cavities. Similarly, recent surveys of liners in North American schools of medicine show no agreement on a standard pulp protection protocol. 38 percent of the 39 schools of dental medicine in the survey reported that calcium hydroxide liner was used for deep cavities filled with amalgam and 30.8% used glass ionomer. The study also reported that for deep composite fillings, the use of glass ionomer was 35.9%, followed by calcium hydroxide at 28.2% [5].

A study by Hilton and Thomas was conducted to examine methods to protect dental pulp among 500 dental students (stagers), young doctors, and doctors at various educational institutions in Pakistan and concluded that contemporary protocols for pulp conservation were not available. Donors respond to the institutions that participated in the survey. For example, approximately 89% of the respondents did not consider the remaining dentin thickness, while 82% of them considered the use of calcium hydroxide as a liner [7].

The objective of this study is, to find out how liners are used in the anterior teeth of the jaws to preserve pulp tissue in patients who have been referred to the dentistry teaching clinic due to dental caries in 2018.

2. Materials and methods

This study is done using the case series and retrospective data methods that were registered. As the patients' registration book of 2018 was reviewed and related cases were recorded in the table prepared for data collection, which was later included in the excel sheet, and finally, the percentage and number of different liner usage, the percentage and number of anterior teeth, the number of liners used according to gender and age, and its figures were presented.

3. Results

This study was performed on 123 cases who were referred to the dentistry teaching clinic in 2018. The results of this study are as follows:

The percentage of liner usage in the age group of 16–30 years old is 73%, in the age group of 31–40 years old is 15%, in the age group of 41–50 years old is 8% and in the age group is 51–65 years is 4%, respectively (**Figure 1**).

This study shows the percentage of liner users is 59.3% for women and 40.7% for men (**Figure 2**).

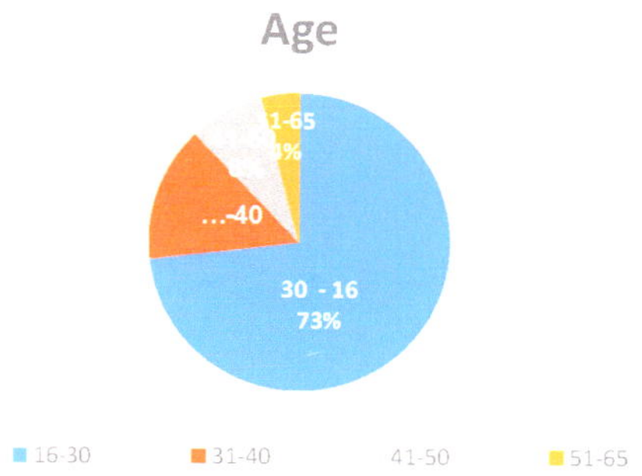

Figure 1.
Shows the percentage of liner usage in the different age groups.

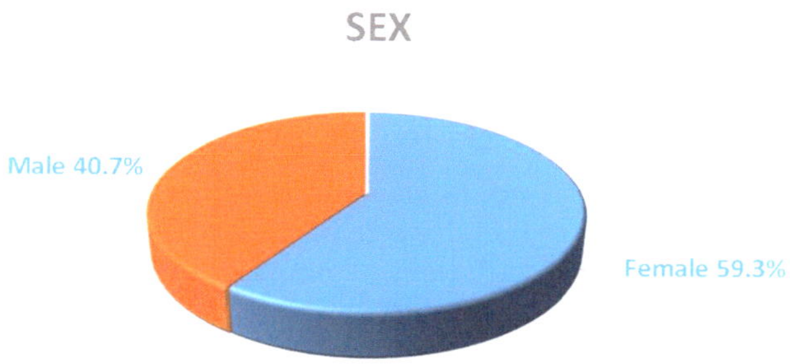

Figure 2.
Shows the use of liners percentage in anterior teeth of upper and lower teeth according to sex.

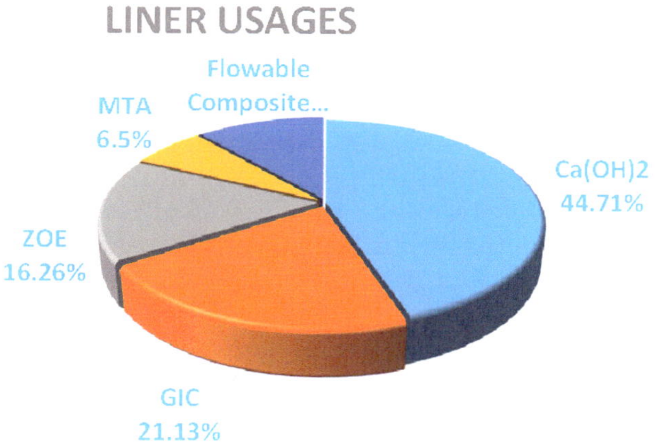

Figure 3.
Shows how to use liners in terms of percentage.

In this study, calcium hydroxide was used in 44.71% of cases, glass ionomer was used in 21.13% of cases, zinc oxide eugenol was used in 16.26% of cases, and a flowable composite was used in 11.38% of cases and MTA was used in 6.5% of cases (**Figure 3**).

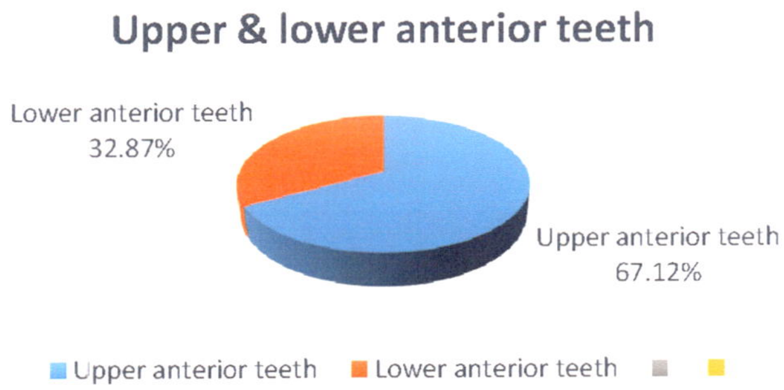

Figure 4.
Shows the percentage of liner use in the anterior of upper and lower teeth.

The percentage of liner use in the maxillary anterior teeth is 67.12% and in the mandibular anterior teeth is 32.87% (**Figure 4**).

4. Discussion

In this study, the different usage of liners in the anterior teeth of the jaws in the dentistry teaching clinic was evaluated. In this study, liners such as Calcium Hydroxide, Glass Ionomer, Zinc Oxide Eugenol, Flowable Composite, and MTA were used in patients who received caries treatment. In this study, the use of liners was evaluated according to the anterior teeth of the upper and lower jaw, sex, and age. Therefore, here it is necessary to compare research findings with the literature. In this study, among the 123 cases that were referred to the dentistry teaching clinic in 2018, in 55 (44.71%) cases, calcium hydroxide was used as a liner, in 26 (21.13%) cases, glass ionomer was used, in 20 (16.26%) cases, zinc oxide eugenol was used, in 14 (11.38%) cases, the flowable composite was used, and in 8 (6.5%) cases, MTA was used as a liner.

The results of pulp cap studies using MTA are encouraging. The following example may help to illustrate this point: "According to the results of the present study and other related studies, MTA is superior to calcium hydroxide for pulp capping of mechanically exposed teeth." In one study, the pulps of 14 teeth were intentionally exposed, half of which were capped with calcium hydroxide and the other half with MTA. The teeth were extracted after one, two, three, four weeks, and six months and evaluated histologically. During the final evaluation period (six months), only one tooth in each group was evaluated. Based on these results, it appeared that MTA was superior to calcium hydroxide [8].

MTA is promising material, but calcium hydroxide indicates a long history of clinical success that MTA cannot currently claim. A review of 14 clinical studies, including more than 2300 cases of calcium hydroxide pulp caps, reported a success rate of up to 90% by experienced physicians. In addition, calcium hydroxide is successful even when done under less-than-ideal clinical conditions. To better elucidate the relative advantages of MTA over calcium hydroxide, prospective clinical trials comparing MTA with calcium hydroxide are required for pulp cap. Research networks based on such a study are engaged [8].

In a human clinical trial, a pulp cap was performed using ZOE. In this study, all pulp capping teeth with ZOE showed chronic inflammation, without pulp healing and dentin bridge formation, up to 12 weeks after the procedure. Conversely, all calcium hydroxide-controlled teeth showed improvement within 4 weeks [8].

Similar to ZOE, a human study of direct pulp cap with glass ionomer showed chronic inflammation and no dentin bridge formation up to 300 days after pulp capping, while calcium hydroxide control groups showed significantly better pulp recovery [8].

In a study conducted by Andreea C Didilescu and colleagues in October 2018 according to Meta-Analysis, they compared the use of MTA and calcium hydroxide in the formation of hard tissue as a barrier (dentin bridge) and suggest that the positive effects of MTA on calcium Hydroxide is better to form hard tissue, and evidence suggests that MTA is more effective than calcium hydroxide in protecting the pulp if the pulp is mechanically exposed [8].

One study showed that the resin composite, as a pulp cap material, showed less pulp healing, chronic inflammation even in the absence of bacteria, and a reduced repair capacity for pulpitis due to dental caries [7].

A study was conducted about pulp capping carious exposures in adults, a randomized controlled trial investigating mineral trioxide aggregate versus calcium hydroxide. The Kaplan–Meier survival analysis showed a cumulative estimate rate of 85% for the MTA group and 52% for the calcium hydroxide group ($P = 0.006$). There was no significant association between the pulp capping material and postoperative pain. Mineral trioxide aggregate performed more effectively than a conventional calcium hydroxide liner as a direct pulp capping material with carious pulpal exposure in adult patients [9].

Mehmet Kemal and Calskan 2017 evaluated MTA pulp capped teeth and demonstrated a slightly higher success rate than calcium hydroxide, it can be recommended as a reliable direct pulp capping material. Direct pulp capping with MTA is a straightforward procedure with a favorable outcome of 24- to 72-month follow-ups in vital mature asymptomatic permanent teeth with carious exposed pulp [10].

A study was conducted about the treatment outcome of mineral trioxide aggregate or calcium hydroxide direct pulp capping for long-term results. The results of this study indicate that MTA provides better long-term results after direct pulp capping compared with calcium hydroxide placing a permanent restoration immediately after direct pulp capping is recommended (odds ratio = 3.18; 95% CI, 1.61–6.3; $P = .004$) [11].

A systematic review and meta-analysis result showed the effect of mineral trioxide aggregate and calcium hydroxide for direct pulp capping is different, as measured by the clinical and radiographic analysis. A statistically significant difference was found between the success rates of MTA and calcium hydroxide-treated teeth that needed direct pulp capping ($P = 0.002$). Clinical assessments of the MTA versus calcium hydroxide for direct pulp capping suggested that MTA was superior to calcium hydroxide in direct pulp capping resulting in a lower failure rate (risk difference 0.1 [95% CI 0.04 to 0.16]). MTA has a higher clinical success rate for direct pulp capping compared to calcium hydroxide and might be a suitable replacement for calcium hydroxide [12].

A study was conducted by Uzay Koc Vural et al. to compare the clinical performance of cavities with no lining and lining with resin-modified glass ionomer for the treatment of root surface carious lesions. The clinical performance of both unlined and RMGI-lined cavities at the 5-year post-restoration assessment was acceptable and there was no significant difference in the clinical performance of the lined and unlined restorations ($P < 0.05$) [13].

S Cushley et al. studied in 2021 the efficacy of direct pulp capping for the management of cariously exposed pulps in permanent teeth. The results were based on poor methodological quality studies. The effect size for MTA vs. calcium hydroxide, low-quality evidence suggests a high success rate for direct pulp capping in teeth with cariously exposed pulps with better long-term outcomes for MTA and Biodentine compared with calcium hydroxide [14].

A study was conducted about outcomes of direct pulp capping by using either ProRoot mineral trioxide aggregate or Biodentine in permanent teeth with carious pulp exposure in 6 to 18-year-old patients. The result shows that Biodentine was non-inferior to ProRoot MTA when used as a direct pulp cap material for cariously exposed permanent teeth of 6 to 18-year-old patients. However, Biodentine did not cause any gray discoloration in this study [15].

A study was conducted to assess the effectiveness of different direct pulp-capping (DPC) materials for human pulp-exposed teeth. An electronic search was performed on 20 February 2018. Long-term clinical and radiographic evaluations of the effectiveness of different DPC materials for use on human pulp-exposed teeth were included. Of the 496 identified articles, 15 met the eligibility criteria. Among the studies included in those articles, a total of 1322 teeth were treated with 12 types of DPC materials, and 1136 teeth were evaluated at a final follow-up examination. For mineral trioxide aggregate (MTA) and calcium hydroxide, the number of included studies, the number of treated teeth, and the mean follow-up period of studies were almost equal, and the success rates of MTA were superior to calcium hydroxide. Therefore, MTA is likely to be a more effective and predictable material for DPC compared to calcium hydroxide [16].

A randomized clinical trial about direct pulp capping with calcium hydroxide, MTA, and Biodentine in permanent young teeth with caries had done. At the follow-up examination at 1 week, the patients showed 100% clinical success. At 3 months, there was 1 failure in the calcium hydroxide group. At 6 months, there were 4 new failures (1 in the calcium hydroxide group and 3 in the MTA group). At 1 year, there was another failure in the calcium hydroxide group. There were no statistically significant differences among the experimental groups. Although no significant differences were found among the materials studied, Biodentine and MTA offered some advantages over calcium hydroxide [17].

Current philosophies and indications for use of cavity sealers, liners, and bases showed that traditional dental education has recommended the generous use of bases and liners under restorations, primarily to prevent postoperative sensitivity. However, new developments in bases and liners, as well as a better understanding of pulp biology, have changed the indications for the use of these materials. Understanding the properties of currently available materials and how they interact with pulpal tissues can help the practitioner decide when to use bases and liners and which products to choose [7].

However, the evaluation conducted in this study shows that the use of MTA liner in comparison to the literature review, in comparison to other liners and its clinical benefits, has been 6.5% (8 cases) in a year, which is very low, and few cases and it is due to the price of MTA that dentistry teaching clinic in Afghanistan as a governmental health sector cannot provide MTA for all cases that need MTA.

5. Conclusion

In this study, calcium hydroxide was used in more cases and MTA was used in fewer cases and it is due to MTA price. The liner usage in the younger age group is more than older age group. This study shows the usage of liners is higher in women than men. The modality liners usage in the maxillary anterior teeth is higher than in the mandibular anterior teeth.

Author details

Husniya Azim* and Shiba Azim
KUMs, Kabul, Afghanistan

*Address all correspondence to: dr.husniya.azim@gmail.com

References

[1] Garg N, Garg A. Textbook of operative dentistry. New Delhi, India: Jaypee Brothers Medical Publishers (P) Ltd.; 2015. pp. 218-221

[2] Arandi NZ. Calcium hydroxide liners: A literature review. Clinical, Cosmetic and Investigational Dentistry. 2017;**9**:67-72

[3] Aggarwal V et al. Effect of flowable composite liner and glass ionomer on class II gingival marginal adaptation of direct composite restorations with different bonding strategies. Journal of Dentistry. 2014;**42**(5):19-25

[4] Hilton TJ. Keys to clinical success with pulp capping: A review of the literature. HHS Author Manuscripts. 2019;**34**(5):615-625

[5] Weiner R. Liners and bases in general dentistry. Australian Dental Journal. 2011;**56**:11-22

[6] Hilton TJ. Keys to clinical success with pulp capping: A review of the literature. HHS Public Access. 2010;**34**(5):615-625

[7] Hilton T. Cavity sealers, liners, and bases: Current philosophies and indications for use. Operative Dentistry. 1996;**21**:46-134

[8] Didilescu AC et al. The effect of dental pulp-capping materials on hard-tissue barrier formation: A systematic review and meta-analysis. American Dental Association. 2018;**249**(10):903-917

[9] Kundzina R et al. Capping carious exposures in adults: A randomized controlled trial investigating mineral trioxide aggregate versus calcium hydroxide. International Endodontic Journal. 2017;**50**(10):924-932

[10] Kemal M, Guneri P. Prognostic factors in direct pulp capping with mineral trioxide aggregate or calcium hydroxide: 2- to 6-year follow-up. Clinical Oral Investigations. 2017;**21**(1):357-367

[11] Mente J et al. Treatment outcome of mineral trioxide aggregate or calcium hydroxide direct pulp capping. Journal of Endodontics. 2014;**40**(11):46-51

[12] Zhu C et al. Clinical outcome of direct pulp capping with MTA or calcium hydroxide: A systematic review and meta-analysis. International Journal of Clinical and Experimental Medicine. 2015;**8**(11):55-60

[13] Vural UK et al. Effect of cavity lining on the restoration of root surface carious lesions: A split-mouth, 5-year randomized controlled clinical trial. Clinical Oral Investigations. 2020;**24**(2):979-989

[14] Cushley S et al. Efficacy of direct pulp capping for management of cariously exposed pulps in permanent teeth: A systematic review and meta-analysis. International Endodontic Journal. 2021;**54**(4):556-571

[15] Parinvaprom N et al. Outcomes of direct pulp capping by using either proroot mineral trioxide aggregate or biodentine in permanent teeth with carious pulp exposure in 6- to 18-year-old patients: A randomized controlled trial. Journal of Endodontics. 2018;**44**(3):341-348

[16] Matsuura T et al. Long-term clinical and radiographic evaluation of the effectiveness of direct pulp-capping materials. Journal of Oral Science. 2019;**61**(1):1-12

[17] Brizuela C et al. Direct pulp capping with calcium hydroxide, mineral trioxide aggregate, and biodentine in permanent young teeth with caries: A Randomized Clinical Trial. Journal of Endodontics. 2017;**43**(11):1776-1780